Killing It

Antony J Stowers

Intro

This is a book for those who smoke and want to stop and for those who've stopped but need reassurance. I'm the latter. I'm never going to take the crown from Allan Carr who has written one of the best 'quit smoking' self-help books the modern world has ever seen, so I wrote this book to bolster my resolve and hopefully help others. Consisting of some cold facts, some home-spun philosophies and some hard life experience, 'Killing It' meanders through time and the history of my promising but ultimately disappointing life in an attempt to understand and fill the void, a void often otherwise stuffed with substance-abuse of one kind or another as I struggled to make sense of it all.

I've also decorated my book with oblique ways of looking at all the associated smoker's paraphernalia, good and bad role models, the 'gateway' hypothesis, various notions around health as well as slavery/freedom viewpoints and interwoven references all as a way of giving context and comparison to the social, economic, emotional, psychological, cultural or environmental states that shape negative choices and poor personal behaviour. But I'm no expert.

Smoking cigarettes was the 'gateway drug' for me in that it did indeed lead to increased drug experimentation and riskier behaviour. When this behaviour affected my destiny and much of the early promise I showed became neglected, chances started to slip by. I could have been a contender but I screwed up, a classic cliché of the age.

Let me tell you why. I make money from teaching my language but I also love acting and producing music – onstage, on film. I still do. But it's too late in life now to make much of it. It just is – trust me. And I didn't fuck it up because I liked acting - I fucked it up because I liked acting very much: I was the right height, size and weight and had a face that suited the screen: blue eyes, a square jaw line, a facial balance with no visible scars and though my teeth weren't perfect, could be. I brushed my hair back to make it spiky or shaved it all off to reveal my strong forehead and I knew how to command presence both on the stage and in a room full of strangers. Lots of other people agreed with my being prime material, some of them wanting to invest in me, represent and promote me. But to do those things – to invest, support and promote – takes trust, trust between them and me. And I couldn't deliver that trust. I couldn't give them what they needed. I fucked it up because I was scared. I didn't really know who I was. They saw that. They could see through me. I thought I knew. I pretended I knew. I adopted different personalities to wear as masks to show to the outside world but I didn't *really* know who I was. I fucked it up because I wasn't mature. Instead of being brave and seeking my hidden cache of courage, I got involved with legal and illegal drugs and drink instead to fill in the ever-widening crevasse not only between me and them but between this pretend person I presented to the world and the real me, almost the as yet unborn me. My life since has been a messy and erratic voyage and in more recent years an increasingly desperate battle to recover scraps of dignity and cushion the inevitable aches and pains that are starting to arrive.

To tame and control my smoking addiction I wracked my brains trying to find a suitable name for 'it' but every time I settled on one I seemed to find some other reason to take it away or change it again as if 'normalising' this insidious thing made it somehow more human, more acceptable. The more I tried to make it more acceptable and thus more reasonable and approachable and able to compromise as humans are supposed to be able to do, the more I realised my resistance stiffened with this prospect and that in fact I could never humanize 'it'. So, winning no prizes for originality, I called 'it' simply It. 'It' would never earn my respect. It should never earn my respect. It doesn't deserve any respect. It doesn't have one name. It doesn't deserve one name. It's changing and twisting and pulling away from me at ever opportunity it can, trying to wriggle free of an arresting grip. It's the least flattering title I dare baptise 'It' with and only by placing a capital I in front of the lowercase t can I separate 'It' from the pronoun used as a substitute for a subject or an object.

So, let's make a deal, or I'll make a deal with you. As long as you're reading this book, you won't smoke. I don't mean just as long as you are physically holding the book in your hands and lifting the words from the page with your eyes. I mean even if you read a little, a few pages, then put it down and go off and do something else and then come back to it again, as long as there is a relationship between you and the contents of this book, you won't smoke. Is that a deal? I mean, sure, you can cheat. You can say yes but have no intention of keeping your promise to me or to yourself. But I was thinking you went for the longer-term option: you don't smoke at all while reading the book but don't re-start again between reading the various chapters and use this 'deal' you and I are making right now as an incentive to read the book as fast as possible, right?

Do you consider yourself a strong person? Are you sure? I'm just checking. Because if you answer yes you are and yet you can't even make a deal as simple as not smoking as long as you're reading this relatively short book, well, I don't want to put words into your head but . . . Maybe when you get to the end you'll be gasping? That's probably going to be the case if you only read to the end of this introductory chapter. I can tell you with 100% certainty you're NOT deciding that for yourself. There's no dignity in slavery. If you want dignity, you've got to be emancipated, freed, liberated or born again.

So did we make the deal? You know what? I'm going to presume we did and that's why you're about to turn the page and read on. And anyway, I don't want you invading my pages with your stinking fumes. If you want to do that, write your own book.

AJS

Chapter Headings

1 – The bill to pay
2 – Quitting is easy
3 – When I was a kid - 1963
4 – The Geneva Convention
5 – Growing Up - 1979
6 – Know your enemy
7 – Losing my cherry - 1982
8 – The E Word
9 – The Leader - 1984
10 – What's yours is mine and what's mine is yours
11 – Poverty in youth - 1985
12 – Smile!
13 - Philosophies of the 80s
14 – A good hockle
15 – Through the gateway
16 – The junkie and his works
17 – Arrival London - 1985
18 - Matches
19 – Rolling papers
20 - A bad groove - 1989-91
21 - Lighters
22 – The Gateway Hypothesis
23 – Life on the run - 1990
24 – Trainspotting - 1992
25 - Dignity by the bootstraps - 1996
26 – The Showdown - 2001
27 – Emigration - 2006
28 – Big Effort - 2009
29 – Relapse - 2010
30 – Stumbling in the city - 2011
31 – And still the battle goes on . . .
32 – D Day - 2012

1 – The bill to pay

I started smoking and taking drugs at the age of about 21. I'm now 51. I was a bit of a late starter, among smokers I mean. There was always kudos to be able to claim to have started smoking at about fourteen or younger while still at school. There still is. When adults boast of how young they were when the started smoking or how often they smoked at a very young age I don't detect shame but instead hear a desperate search for a compliment or at least that I should be impressed.

But I didn't start until I was 21. I'd left home the year before but as my parents hadn't smoked nor taken drugs and because in the first place I lived in after leaving home the landlady didn't smoke or take drugs, I continued in that vein. But as soon as I started hanging out with influential peers and then started to share my next home with one of those people, Chris, ten years older than me and who already smoked and took drugs in copious amounts, as did the circle of friends he mixed with and who quickly became my friends and part of my social circle, I succumbed to the temptation.

I managed to seriously (but temporarily) quit smoking twice for a combined total of about three years so, give or take, that's still about 25 years of caning my body with tobacco and drugs.

Going backwards from today I quit smoking on May 30th 2012. I'd restarted September 17th 2010 after a break of about 18 months. There was then a long period of about 8 years going back to 2002 when I'd managed to stay away from both dope and tobacco for about 18 months. That took me back to February 2000 and prior to that I hadn't stopped smoking since 1984.

How much did I spend? No idea. A wild estimate based on an even £2 a day for twenty-five years on tobacco must be about £16,000 at 2017 prices. I also smoked dope, marijuana or hashish, mostly hashish, and spent almost £2.5K on dope in 2012/2013 alone but that was close to the end when it was getting out of control. The main delivery system of both of those drugs is still by mixing it with tobacco, usually the rolled variety as it burns down at a slower rate. Even £10 a month for a year would be £120 per annum x by 25 years and would make £3000 but it was much more than £10 a month, so double it and half that and add it all up and it still only comes to a conservative £6.5K. That's a lot of money to somebody who never had much.

So even this conservative calculation of nicotine consumption, when added to an almost unknown estimate or dope consumption, might work out at about £25,000 over 28 years but I've no way of being accurate – no receipts, no legal transactions and no refunds.

I rarely act anymore in anything but amateur dramatic productions and keep myself fed and lodged and functioning in this world with a mixture of state welfare and teaching. This also keeps my brain active. Would it function better today if I hadn't taken so many drugs yesterday? There's a question. My hair is grey but then at 51 maybe that would have happened anyway? I've got slightly more weight around my middle but that's because I eat too much and don't do enough exercise to compensate, having relied on tobacco as an appetite suppressant for 30 years. My teeth aren't in great condition, partly because of the calcium deficiency I had when I was a kid but mostly because cigarette smoking and then cigarette-replacement substances (like coffee) have stained them.

I'm not making any claims to be a medical expert. I'm often paraphrasing or re-phrasing information taken from elsewhere and my only 'expertise' in this sad affair is comparing this newer information with my own experiences. Nonetheless, I have to write frankly and in doing so expose my own vulnerability and stupidity (lack of intelligent choices) to complete strangers – that's possibly you, family, friends and journalists, but hey, you knew already, right?

My ignorance was based on how little I knew or how little I was told before I entered into experimentation with a particular drug. We had no Internet back then, no rapid way to access vast and up-to-date arsenals of information. We only had rumours, lurid newspaper reports or vague threats that 'Smoking will kill you' and getting facts was difficult.

I thought I'd made the choice to be an on-and-off addict for thirty years but I never seemed to be able to get my head out of the mist long enough to see that in fact the drugs and the addictions made the choice for me - I was just along for the ride.

Despite being a few kilos overweight, I'm now illegal and legal drug-free but I'm not out of the woods – the search for dopamine, melatonin and endorphins, the natural 'reward' chemicals which are activated when I sense natural pleasures like eating food I like, is constant.

Even the definition of 'drug' as a noun and as a verb needs to be reinforced so it doesn't become a just another item accepted into our language without consequence. The Little Oxford Dictionary of Current English (sitting here on my bookshelf) says that as a noun it is a 'medicinal substance, esp. pain-killer, stimulant, narcotic etc, and as a verb to 'administer drugs to; indulge in narcotics etc.' A narcotic is classed as an adjective 'inducing drowsiness, sleep, or insensibility' or 'medicinally administered drowsiness'.

'Medicinally administered drowsiness' first entered my life around the age of 20, in 1984, and finally left my life – or I finally rejected it – in December 2013, so it really was the best part of 30 years, on and off.

If you ask most people why they started smoking cigarettes they'll most likely tell you what I'm telling you now – because your friends did it or because you thought it was cool. Obviously you can start at any age. You can't argue that only weak people smoke – many extremely brave and adventurous people smoke. War heroes smoked! So you can't argue that to smoke means to be weak. It's a certain type of weakness or we have to then argue that people are strong for some things and weaker for other things and in different ways.

I was 18 years old in 1981, unemployed and living in a God-forsaken town called Middlesbrough in the county of Cleveland in north east England and still living at home. It would be easy to say that these external economic and social forces cornered me into low self-esteem and thus into bad habits like smoking and drinking to escape from that reality, but there were plenty amongst our neighbours who also suffered from economic, political and social pressure who didn't turn to smoking and drinking or escape. Neither of my parents smoked and my younger brother was only a baby and none of my four grandparents smoked, apart from Grandad Jack – my Dad's Dad – he smoked a pipe.

For as long as I remember he'd smoked a pipe. He happily sat in front of a coal fire in his living room puffing away at his pipe while watching cricket on television. In the days when coal and coke fires were popular, it seemed a bit pointless to complain about the relatively small amount of cigarette and pipe smoke in the air compared with the millions of chimneys, industrial furnaces, power station chimneys and steam engines pumping out millions of tons of CO_2 every day. It's only in recent times, as we've switched radically away from smokeless fuels, that cigarette and tobacco smoke have at last been isolated, cornered almost until we can smother it completely.

As a kid in those days I happily accepted without question or judgement Grandad's right to sit in his own house and fill the air with tobacco smoke fumes. It wasn't something anybody objected to, it was just accepted. It would never have occurred to anyone to suggest he went outside in fact it would have been classed as an insult! As *kids* we were always made aware that smoking was very much an adult past-time and it was forbidden for us, but I think that habit has been eternal, the idea of certain things being forbidden to kids that are allowed to adults. I was lucky in that my parents didn't smoke in the home so I never grew up with it but a lot of my friends' parents smoked and I guess they too must have just assumed it was acceptable. I'm sure quite a few didn't, many hated it and thought it disgusting but very few would have objected.

Until the age of 14, I grew up in a two-bedroom brick terraced house with no garden ringed by cobbles and pavements. These were homes for the working class. The general association for the working class is the connection between their background and education and borderline poverty. I wouldn't claim we wore rags and starved to death but there was certainly a lack of luxuries. The case is still the same today and it can be argued that a difficult existence can be made more palatable by drinking and smoking. But again we're going back to that post-war lifestyle whereby virtually everyone was poorly educated to high-fat foods or diseases associated with smoking and excessive drinking. My mother smoked when she was carrying me in the womb and then later in adult life I seemed more responsive to it. Coincidence?

2 - Quitting is easy

So you've stocked up on coffee, chocolates and DVD's, locked the door and told all your friends you're not to be disturbed. You've reserved a quiet weekend in the comfort of your own home and sent the kids away to visit relatives, or maybe booked yourself in at a retreat or a cheap hotel. You've thrown the ashtrays in the bin, along with the lighters. You either smoked the last cigarette in the box or the final wisp of rolling tobacco in the pouch and you made sure there are no more skins lying around. All other events had been cancelled and you went to the local pharmacy or chemists' shop and, after consulting with the assistant and reading the instructions, applied the 11mg Nicotine Patches to your skin by rolling up your sleeve, sticking one on your inner lower arm where there's a nice thick vein and rolling your sleeve back down again. Somewhere in your mind there's a voice that says this gives you a feeling of relief but you don't know if it's going to be as effective as that familiar habit of putting a paper tube between your lips and sucking in. Your hands and fingers feel liberated of a sudden. After only an hour you feel different, stronger than you did one hour before. So you put on your best walking boots and coat and set out for a long walk that'll take most of the afternoon to complete, filling your lungs with fresh air so you can get a good long march going, aware that every breath and ever step is flushing out the carcinogens and replacing them with oxygen. You take a longer and more circuitous route than normal and after a while you wonder why you didn't do this walking business more often? As you march along the beach or through the forest, you start to think about your friends and family who lectured you for so long about your pitiful addiction, how they'd now pat you on the back if they could see you now and tell you how proud they are. Like a soldier, you'll beat a rhythm in your head with a brisk 'Left-Left, Left, Right, Left' and think about everything and anything that takes your mind off your affliction. Eventually, you'll get back home and the first thing you'll do is make yourself a nice cup of sweet tea and then find a nice chair and sit in it and drink it and, probably more exhausted than you've been for a while, lay down to sleep as long as you can. You might go up close to the mirror, smile and examine your smile in the reflection but despair at their colour and the grey of your gums and give them another thorough scrub. When you wake up, you might cough a few times to clear your throat and spit out the filth, then look down at your lower arm and wonder if you should have followed the instructions on the box to the letter and taken off the patch to sleep? But seeing as it was your first day and night, you left it on with the conviction that as long as it sat there you felt strong and as long as you feel strong and master of this situation, you were in with a chance. You still are – even as you shower you make sure no water touches the patch to loosen the gum that keeps it on your porous skin. That's when you realise you've gone one full day, twenty-four hours, without feeding It. When was the last time in our life you had the courage to go one full day without It? With a heavy heart and some distress you realise you have *never* gone one full day without nicotine probably since you started. You can even remember your life before, as a kid growing up or as a teenager, how happily and freely you lived and existed and worked and played and suffered and struggled through all the nitty-gritty details of human existence. You dealt with every single blow with aplomb or stoicism and never once did it cross your mind that smoking a cigarette would bring you the gratifying answer to your problem that you sought. Remember how it was before? Yes, you just got on with it. You dealt with it. Remember that? That was you. You did that once. And you can do it again. You spend Day Two wading through your DVD's and chocolates. Oh sure, you've heard all the stories of how people quitting start\eating and putting on weight but somehow you feel that's a small price to pay for your addiction and anyway, you tell yourself, would I be stuffing all this stuff into my face unless my body wasn't trying to tell me how hungry it had been all those years? Eating is just your body's way of dealing with hunger. Of course the outside world sticks its unwanted head into your business, there's no real avoiding it these days. You want to proudly tell a friend or two how you've quit smoking but something holds you back maybe because, somewhere deep, deep down inside, they want you to fail. You don't want to put pressure on yourself. Non-smokers, people who've never smoked, they won't do that. They'll support you all the way down the line. But smokers and even some ex-smokers, but particularly smokers without the courage to quit, they'll be envious and the Beast they have inside of them, their version of 'It', will be feeding doubts, lies and tricks into their minds

Monday morning will arrive. You've removed the old patch and put on a new one. Although tiny in comparison to the rest of you, you feel protected by this little thing as if it was a space age gadget covering and hiding your entire body by some invisible cloak from whatever damage may be rained down on you by evil aliens trying to stun you with their death waves. A long week will stretch ahead. You may have to finally leave the protection of your little secret world. You'll see them within minutes, maybe seconds: pathetic addicts walking along smoking or standing around smoking as if their stupid habit makes the quality of their moment somehow more satisfying. You'll rush past waving your hand to disperse the exhaled smoke. Pity them but take heart from the fact that you're now into Day Three and you're doing okay. Two days without! When was the last time you went for two days without? Ten years ago? Twenty? More? You're a New Man or a New Woman. You'd forgotten how strong and courageous you could be.

You'd always suspected it but you'd never had the courage to find out. "Tomorrow" you'd always lied "Tomorrow I'll be a hero!" Well tomorrow finally caught up with you and called in its loan and to your great surprise you put your hands in your pocket and pulled them out again - payment in full. You want your arm to reach out around and pat yourself on the back for a job well done. More challenges will lie ahead but you've proved to yourself you CAN go whole days without. Wouldn't it be great if you could turn two days into three and three into four and four into five and this time next Monday you'll realise you'll have gone a whole week without? The addiction will have been cut – it only takes a few days, it says so on the box and in all the guides. You'll keep the patches on, of course. You'll take no chances. You won't tempt fate. As long as that little sticker is on your arm you are protected. 'It' is waiting for you, standing in the background drumming its fingers patiently on the table top and sneering at you with disdain, just knowing you're going to crack and let It back in again and then It's going to put a rotten arm around you and whisper in your ear: "See? I told you so!" After a week though It will start to get irritated and once you start coughing up the vile black mucus from your lungs and It has you crippled over with a hernia trying to hack it out of yourself, then it'll be dancing on your back shouting: "Why are you doing this to yourself? Why? Haven't I always kept you safe and comfortable through your dark hours, occupying your impatient hands and fingers, to make you look cool and seem like a risk-talker in front of friends and strangers?"

You'll notice the improvements in subtle ways and reasonably quickly in the first month – your sense of smell will return, as will your sense of taste. You'll notice how your clothes, car interior if you have one or home interior, which I'm presuming you do have, will clear up. You'll be coughing up some really vile stuff from your lungs by now, almost on a daily basis and usually more first thing in the morning. You'll probably have put on weight a little but not excessively. Remember: this is just what you and millions of other non-smokers who try to watch what their diets do. Smokers eat less, a lot less. Eating more is just normal, not indulgent. Your body is recovering from the years of draining it of all the usual vitamins, proteins, fibre and magnesium that It has robbed it of for years. For all those years, It was like those rotten soldiers who steal from the Red Cross parcels meant for prisoners. Chances are that by now you're off the patches too. They're all used up and the box has gone in the bin. Maybe you bought some more, maybe you didn't. Either way it's a month now and the worst is over. If you can do one month, you can do two months.

You've probably lost a 'friend' or two, smokers of course. They won't want to be near you because they won't have the courage to do what you're doing and they won't want to be reminded of their lack of courage by having you around. No, they'll want to be on their own or with other smokers. You may even have lost a loved one because they're probably or possibly also addicted but show no signs of supporting you. You'll have to make that choice for them. Their fear, ignorance and lack of any convincing argument to the contrary will dispirit, depress and distress you to the point of despair and maybe even provoke anger and separation. But this is what it takes to be free of It. It will be getting really crazy by now, trying to convince you that you can't stand around at a bus stop or in a public space without smoking, fooling yourself into believing it somehow makes the time pass more rapidly or that those moments are better. And even if the worst came to the worst and you were stupid enough to let It in via the back door, you know you've given yourself a one month break and the world didn't end. You avoided drinking too much because it might have broken down your resistance. You laugh at the ridiculousness of your workmates constantly sneaking outside or going to the toilets to have a crafty puff or two because they don't have the courage or sense to see how they are being controlled, telling themselves they're exercising rational choice and enjoying the experience but of course they're simply maintaining the nicotine levels in the bloodstream. As soon as those levels start to drop they need to be replenished. It's a vicious circle but you personally have taken an axe and smashed and broken the chain.

Yep, that was the easy part, quitting. Now comes the tricky bit – staying off.

3 – When I was a kid – 1963

My understanding of cigarettes was formed only by the taboo that was associated with them and I was constantly told: 'Don't smoke' but in the late 1960's and early 1970's cigarettes didn't have aggressive health warnings and there was little understanding or, if there was, little desire to speak about it in public. The NHS dealt with millions of smokers who self-inflicted all manners of horrors on their trusting bodies through passive and secondary smoking in less enlightened times. At a young age I was convinced that even one puff of a cigarette would kill me but of course logic overruled when I saw people weren't falling down dead all around me. The working classes are/were largely associated with drinking and smoking as vices and these became stereotypical. That's not to say tobacco addiction knows class barriers - it doesn't but somehow I could never envisage wine bars and cocktail parties full of people puffing away on Embassy fags while clutching pints of bitter. Spirits like whisky, vodka, gin and brandy weren't associated with working class recreation, at least not on a daily basis. The preferred drink in those days was bitter, lager and cider, always in pint or half-pint glasses. In my parents' world spirits were associated with alcoholism and reserved for hardened drinkers. If it was Christmas or a birthday somebody might have a nip of 'something stronger' but I honestly think drinking pints was to do with socialising. It takes much longer to drink a pint of bitter than it does to drink a shot of whisky or gin or vodka. Spirits in small glasses, even mixed with lemonade or orange, weren't considered 'manly' in those days.

The culture that revolved around working class recreation and working class social and drinking lifestyle perpetuated for centuries: men working in hard, physical and often monotonous jobs needing liquid relief. Today microchips have overtaken or replaced the repetitive tasks but people of my father's generation spent their entire working lives in overalls, working in dirty and often dangerous conditions, in hot weather or cold, day and night. My Dad must have spent half of his 50 year working life on night shifts. Social drinking, sport – as much as betting on horses was considered sport - and television were the outlets for millions of working class people because wages were pegged to low-paid and often low-skilled jobs, there wasn't a lot of extra money to spare on drinking. Beer was the same price as spirits but beer in a pint glass lasted longer than spirits in a small glass.

The British high street has been transformed from what it was 30 years ago, as has the British pub. When I was a teenager in the early 1980's going out to pubs was considered to be the *only* thing to do. We all did it. Millions and millions of people geared up their entire lives to the weekend. I'm not sure that's the case anymore since the rise of sport and fitness in daily life, the banning of smoking and online home entertainment. There was a lot of experimentation before the public ban on smoking came into place – restaurants and bars cordoned off certain sections of their spaces to Smokers and Non-Smokers, but as there were no physical walls between the spaces it didn't make a lot of difference. It was more about getting people used to the idea hat smoking was being gradually isolated I suppose.

When, in 1985, I moved to London, one job that sustained me for the first three years and then a further seven years after that was working in pubs, as well as socialising in them. My first real part-time job in London was in a pub near Victoria Park in Hackney, called The Falcon and Firkin, one of a chain that played with the assonance of the F so there were others like The Ferret and Firkin, and so on, themed under birds or animals and spread across London. Not only did they serve well-known brand names but also their own house-brewed bitters, cold food and occasionally cooked dinners. When I first started working there in 1985 there was no concept of one part of the bar being for smokers and the other not, it was all the same. There were no carpets on the floor, only floorboards, so it always had a rough and ready feel, but it wasn't logical anyway to have carpets in bars as they were so many spilled drinks and used cigarettes and residual cigarette ash.

A particular item on the list of the barman in those days was the 'cigarette break', if you smoked it was a slight pause from being on one's feet pulling and serving drinks for hours at a time whereby you'd light up and by the time you'd smoked it down to the butt, start work again. Or you'd grab a bucket and a wet cloth and go from table to table tipping the contents of ashtrays into the bucket, wiping out the ash and then putting it back. It seems amazing now looking back that we lived and played in such an excessive way, literally smoking ourselves to death, but we did.

4 - The Geneva Convention

Until I looked into it, I thought the 'Geneva Convention' was one agreement made by a number of nations regarding the treatment of POW's or Prisoners of War because I heard the term bandied about in war movies or media news. What I discovered is that there were FOUR treaties, or conventions. In 1949 and prior to that there were two international treaties in 1929 and then the first convention in 1864. So when you hear the two words 'Geneva' and 'Convention' used together you should be in theory hearing them in their plural form but for some reason many people use the singular term.

The 1864 convention came about directly because of the creation of the Red Cross and that in turn came into being because of one Henry Dunant, a Swiss businessman who visited wounded soldiers after the Battle of Solferino in 1859. Shocked, disgusted and revolted by the way in which not only wounded but prisoners of war were treated in callous and inhumane ways, he wrote a bestselling *exposé* about his experience called 'A Memory of Solferino', published in 1862. This in turn prompted the creation of the Red Cross, a neutral organisation designed to provide aid to those in need of it during warfare and a protective treaty for its staff. Then came the first international treaty in 1864 in which a definition to 'define the basic rights of wartime prisoners and establish protection for the wounded and sick in and around war zones' was established. Only twelve nations signed up at the beginning so attempts were made in 1906 and 1968 to improve the 1864 conventions, extending protection to those in warfare at sea as well as on land.

Two new 'conventions' were added to the 1929 treaties: one was the third attempt to replace the 'Convention for the amelioration of the condition of the wounded and the sick in armies in the field' of 1864 with a more updated definition and the other came out of the experiences of World War One when it was shown that many of the original ideas in the 1864 were impractical. The Fourth Geneva Convention of 1949 was inspired by the war crimes exposed at the Nuremburg Trials and a new but complicated convention was added 'relative to the Protection of Civilian Persons in Time of War'.

Two more protocols were added in 1977 that extended the terms of the 1949 Conventions with additional protections and in 2005 a third protocol established the addition of a protective sign – the red crystal – for medical services and staff as an alternative to the red cross and red crescent symbols as some countries found these objectionable.

So, to roughly sum up: the first convention dealt with the treatment of wounded and sick armed forces in the field. The second convention dealt with the sick, wounded, and shipwrecked members of armed forces at sea. The third convention dealt with the treatment of prisoners of war during times of conflict and the fourth convention dealt with the treatment of civilians and their protection during wartime.

The various sub-sections and finer details of the conventions are thorough and detailed and make fascinating reading for those who are not fully aware of all they imply and I'd recommend they were read or looked into. I'm certainly not making light of their importance. But in the context of a book about stopping smoking, their main inclusion in this chapter is to help the reader understand that nicotine addiction, cigarettes (in whatever shape or form they take) and those who cultivate, harvest, cure, package, manufacture and sell this product did NOT sign any of the Geneva Conventions. Not one. Addiction and nicotine addiction does NOT take ANY prisoners and does not distinguish between age, sex or rank. It cuts right across the entire swathe of all categories with one cruel stroke and - mark my words - it will NEVER give you a break. Like a parasite, it will cling on to you without remorse, without compromise, without emotion. It will effectively use you as its host body in which It can strengthen it's close contact with you every single minute of every single hour. Time and time again It will remain cold every time, tricking you into thinking you're exercising free will when in fact you surrendered your free will the very first moment you first permitted It to enter your life.

5 – Growing up - 1979

Young working class men and women in the 1970s were still expected to follow in their parents' steps. When I was coming up to my sixteenth birthday I knew I'd shortly be leaving school and going into full-time employment in a shipyard as an apprentice welder and end up a qualified welder like my Dad, or full-time unemployment. Middlesbrough, which was where I grew up, was then famous for shipbuilding and engineering because or the iron ore to be found in the hills around Cleveland. But if our Dad wore a shirt and tie or you had a garden you were considered upper working class or even middle class and pertaining to a university education.

In The Bridge public house, directly opposite the factory gates of Dorman's Shipbuilders and Heavy Engineering, half the men blew their lolly every Friday and Saturday night and some into Sunday. The Bridge often had live bands at the weekends and these places were PACKED to bursting. You often couldn't get in. Queues for the bar were two or three deep. You fought to attract the attention of the bar staff. Some of the busiest bars had bouncers but they were only really there to stop fights developing, unlike today where they seem to have gone one-step further and pre-judgement mode. In my youth lively groups or drinkers were considered good business but now they're considered anti-social.

I fell in with the long hair crowd – hippies and bikers and lovers of drinking and heavy rock. We mixed live rock bands or rock deejays with excessive drinking and smoking, more often than not in extremely small and poorly ventilated cellar spaces. The breweries that sold beer and lager in those days knew that a few pints at the weekend was what most people looked forward to so the prices they charged were proportionately linked with the wages paid. The average price of a pint of beer in Britain in 1979 (the year I left school and started working) was between 20p – 40p, amazing compared with today's prices of anything between £2 and £3! But then again of course the average weekly wage of a working, unskilled man was anything between £60 - 100 a week. In those days wages were mostly paid weekly on Fridays and in cash, so life was set on a regular weekly cycle and at weekends it, your night out, was always in the air and in general conversation.

Homebrew was also an added addition to many homes in those days and probably still is. I remember my Dad dabbled a few times but drinking average-quality cloudy pints at home wasn't the same as drinking clear, stronger volume pints in the conviviality of a pub. I never ever recall seeing a pint of crystal clear home brew in a pint glass brewed either by my Dad or by friends. I only remember pints of cloudy sludge and we were often so impatient we'd drink the sludge as well.

Packets of ten and twenty cigarettes were pegged at about 50p – 55p a packet in 1979.

My first weekly wage was £15. £5 was paid to my parents. 'Paying your board' was, and still is in many families, part of the transition from childhood to adulthood, becoming equipped with the self-discipline needed to cope with living on their own. That left me the princely sum of £10 to spend on myself. £10 doesn't sound like a lot but it only had to tide me over until the following Friday and then I'd get paid again. We'd get our wage packets handed out to us by the Foreman. The girls in the office had filled in our wage slips in pen and ink, stuffed our money in notes and dirty coins into a small brown envelope with our names on. I usually bought one or sometimes two 12' vinyl LP's of rock groups of the day, new jeans or boots every few months and the rest of the money went down the various pubs in Middlesbrough, or sometimes we'd take a bus or a train to nearby Darlington, the railway town, at the weekends. Even after buying the new LP by Kiss or AC/DC at about £2.99, I still had £7 left to spend on pints of lager or cider.

The general idea was to use the long-lasting pint as a social prop to either talk to your mates or chat up a girl or to try and get drunk. With even a maximum average price of 40p a pint, it was theoretically possible to go out on both Friday and Saturday nights and drink about 5 pints each night and have something left over to buy some chips on the way home. I didn't have extra expenses like cars to worry about as I didn't drive and it was a small town so walking home or walking to work was easy. Five pints of lager in one night was quite a lot and the aim was pure and simple really: get drunk or get laid. Getting drunk was associated with being an adult. There was always (and still is today) this period of transition as you shed the trappings of youth like certain unfashionable items of clothing and put on new fashions that you think will portray you in the eyes of other adults as an adult yourself, as if in that transition you suddenly adopt a new personality.

My cousin Joe lived nearby and was a couple of years younger. Separated from each other we were probably quite reasonable kids but when put together we created an entirely new chemistry, egging each other on, pitting our risk-taking skills the one against the other in a kind of youthful game of chance. It was Joe who first introduced me to 'Honey Rose' cigarettes. He knew where they could be legally bought by kids under 16 (in a health food shop near Albert Park) because they contained no tobacco. They were in fact dried, purple-coloured leaves of various non-addictive plants. Back in those days they were considered to be the closest thing available to what we today call the 'electronic' cigarette.

They tried to do the job of the nicotine patch, used as a non-addictive prop to wean oneself off tobacco. They were cheap to buy and came in packs of 20 but when smoked produced huge amounts of scented, blue smoke and tasted vile. When Joe was only 12 and me not much above 14, we bought a packet of 'Honey Rose' and sneaked off to the Municipal Park where we hid among the bushes and secretly lit our cigarettes. Joe smoked most of his and tried to look cool with this white stick doing its damnedest to look casual between his fingers but I didn't inhale it into my lungs because I didn't know how to. A little while later, again out of naïve desperation, I rolled some dried leaves from a tree in the park into a crumbled pile and tried to make a cigarette out of the powder using a sheet of writing paper. Needless to say once the flame of the match hit the end it went up in a whoosh and the leaf powder fell out everywhere. It was lucky it did or I'd have died of a coughing fit.

And that was it, for about five or six years cigarettes remained on the fringes of my life.

6 - Know your enemy

Tobacco is a plant of the nightshade family. There are more than 70 species and the most potent is *nicotina rustica,* indigenous to North and South America, Australia, South West Africa and the South Pacific.

The English word originates from the Spanish and Portuguese word 'tabaco' but the precise origin was said to refer either to the *tabago,* a kind of Y-shaped pipe for sniffing – not inhaling - the smoke.

It was brought to Europe after Columbus's 1492 voyage and soon became one of the chief exports of the southern United States until replaced by cotton – both founded on the back of slavery. We talk in these times of 'globalisation' as if it was a new thing but the farming of tobacco unleashed this phenomenon on the world as far back as the 17th century. In many cases, the natives indigenous to the Americas were not suited to the back-breaking toil of outdoor agriculture and so the great powers colluded and created a triangle between stolen slaves from Africa, their distribution in Europe and transportation to the Americas by a strong Navy and Merchant Marine. They then developed their maritime talents to connect Africa to the Americas. Slaves, when locked up on slaving ships, were actively encouraged to smoke in order to cope with the misery of their incarceration.

After the American Civil War, James Bonsack designed and built a machine that automated cigarette production thus making nicotine delivery rapid, easy, efficient and 'clean' but only in the sense of not involving carrying the paraphernalia around to construct a makeshift delivery system. The invention of matches made access to fire much easier too.

Curing methods vary: sun-cured, air-cured, fire-cured and flue-cured each produce more of less nicotine. Tobacco production requires the use of up to 16 separate pesticides just between planting the seeds and transplanting the young plants to the field. These pesticides and fertilizers end up in the soil, waterways and food chain. Tobacco extracts nutrients such as phosphorus, nitrogen and potassium from the soil more quickly than any other major crop. This leads to dependence on fertilizers and the wood used to cure tobacco in some places leads to deforestation - Brazil uses the wood of 60 million trees per year for curing, packaging and rolling cigarettes. Is it replaced? Are trees replanted at the same rate they are harvested? Who knows?

It's important to remember the 'first-time smoke'. With a first-time smoke – the first few puffs - the initial feeling is of wanting to vomit, lead-heavy legs and a dizziness in the head and behind the eyes but once over this temporary barrier – not puking, forcing the body to maintain - the body stops rejecting. This is because cigarette smoke contains over FOUR THOUSAND chemical compounds, the most well-known and most lethal of which are nicotine and carbon monoxide (a gas formed by the incomplete combustion of the carbon). At least 50 of these compounds are carcinogenic (cancer causing). Harmful effects derive from the different chemicals in the smoke including cyanide, formaldehyde, paraffin, cadmium, nickel, arsenic, tobacco-specific nitrosamines (TSNA's) and phenols.

Nicotine acts on receptors in the brain and CNS (central nervous system) that artificially stimulate release of natural biological compounds such as dopamine and glutamate. Additional chemicals in the blend simply increase this feeling of 'reward' that comes in anticipation of a nicotine boost that is soon to be delivered. This is the 'positive' feeling a smoker has when just about to light a cigarette and deliver nicotine into the bloodstream.

Under Sharia Law, the consumption of cigarettes by Muslims is prohibited.

Uncorroborated studies (rumours) say some tobacco companies have manipulated packaging designs to give the impression the tar level is low but in fact the components and chemical additives are the same as high tar cigarettes, it is simply that the suggestion of lower tar is subtle. Check out 'The Insider' with Al Pacino and Russell Crowe.

A key ingredient that makes cigarettes more addictive is the inclusion of reconstituted tobacco, which has additives to make it burn rapidly. Blending offers a consistent taste that may otherwise change according to environmental and climate conditions for each harvest. The processing produces by-products such as leaf stems, tobacco dust, and tobacco leaf pieces so to improve profits these are processed separately into forms where they can then be added back into the blend without an apparent or marked change in the cigarette's quality. Ammonium is added to the paper to make the cigarette a more effective 'delivery system'. Many of the chemicals simply boost the addictive properties of cigarettes, especially when burned. Ammonia, for example, converts bound nicotine molecules in smoke into free nicotine molecules.

The common name for the remains of a cigarette after smoking is a cigarette butt. The butt makes up 30% of the cigarette's length. Exterior disposed cigarette butts are transported through drains to streams, rivers and beaches. Cigarette filters are the most common form of litter in the world as approximately 5.6 trillion cigarettes are smoked every year worldwide. Of those, an estimated 4.5 trillion cigarette filters become litter. The estimated waste from filters is based on an average pack containing twenty cigarettes makes up an accumulated weight of 3.4 grams for the filters (or butts) alone. On average, each day 15 billion cigarettes are smoked which makes a combined weight of 2.5 million kilos. On an annual basis this makes a staggering 7.65 million (7.65 metric tonnes) kilos of butts.

During my time as a nicotine addict, I smoked Amber Leaf, Benson & Hedges, Camel, Chesterfield, Dunhill, Embassy, Fortuna, Gauloise, Golden Virginia, Gold Leaf, Kent, Lambert & Butler, Lucky Strike, Marlboro, Mayfair, Pall Mall, Peter Stuyvesant, Philip Morris, Senior Service, Woodbine, Winston. Sometimes I alternated according to price, sometimes to availability and other times out of choice.

7 – Losing my cherry - 1982

When I was growing up in the 1970s and 1980s (I was an adult in the 1980s but even in my 20's there was still a sense of 'growing up') there was almost zero information available about drugs. There were books but you had to go to a local library or bookshop and then trawl laboriously through the right ones looking for facts, information and case studies – if you could be bothered. The possession and purchasing of such literature just wasn't part of everyday culture. It wasn't available at the touch of a finger on a keyboard. Back then we survived on rumours, myths, crappy bland b&w photos and evidence we gathered through experience and others. Doctors told us certain things were bad so we believed them because they were educated people, but it didn't necessarily mean people we knew and loved died instantly the moment they stuck a cigarette in their mouths. We saw that didn't happen. So we blindly rolled the dice of risk and hoped when the die stopped spinning on their corners on the slippery tabletop, our numbers would come up marked SAFE or LIFE and not DANGER or DEATH.

I sometimes wonder if it would have changed anything for me even if I'd had had this knowledge back then? Impulse, risk and danger seem to be part of the metabolic make up of humanity.

In 1982 I was 18 and had been out of work for six months, having been made redundant with a year of my apprenticeship left to run. I had no idea what to do, the regular structure of the five-day week, day shift or night shift with options for overtime thrown in was gone.

I'd saved some money, not much, and decided to hitch hike to southern Spain to try to find a job in a hotel but got as far as Calais and then decided to come back to England and hitch hike around until my money ran out. Just before leaving the ferry in Dover, I went to the Duty Free and bought myself 10 boxes of 'Gauloise', the cheapest cigarettes I could find at that time, un-tipped and in distinctive sky blue packets. Again, if I asked myself why I would do something so out of character I'd have to say because I made an association with smoking being somehow 'cool' and by being seen smoking I'd attract other smokers, using the cigarette as a kind of social prop. But Gauloises' un-tipped, hard, choking smoke was unlikely to make me many new friends though it did lend me an air of the exotic.

For the following two weeks I hitched around England, mostly the north and the Lake District, treating myself now and again to what I thought was a kind of pleasure of a cigarette as I strolled by lakes or waited by the sides of roads for lifts. I don't recall getting addicted, despite smoking just about all two hundred of them. By the time my journey came to an end in the last week of May, they'd all been either smoked or shared with people I'd met on the way. I'd experimented. I had no withdrawal symptoms though I noticed nobody ever accepted my offer to give my French ciggies away!

Cigarettes didn't enter my life again until about 1983, largely because of the company I started keeping. I'd spent from November 1981 to November 1983 living with my non-smoking family and living on dole money so I'd never had anything to spare to spend on anything remotely resembling a luxury. Cigarettes fell into that category.

Once I left home that financial situation didn't change. If anything it worsened because I now had to feed myself from the money doled out to me by the government. Life was so unfair! When I'd lived at home I'd eaten what the family ate. When you leave home you of course win a certain heady freedom – you no longer have to tiptoe around the feelings of those with whom you've strong emotional relationships. Living in the attic of a family house - my first bed-sit after leaving home - I still had to consider the needs of the new family who lived below but whatever I'd got away with in the family home was now impossible and no emotional coercion was going to work. It would in fact be turned back onto me as an embarrassing and clumsy tactic.

A lot of people I knew at that time were in much the same position, caught in that strange limbo between teenager and adult, neither too much of one nor too little of the other. We could drink, drive, smoke, vote and have sex legally, but it's better to do those things as a fully mature adult aware of the consequences or at least able to wring maximum pleasure or thrill or efficiency out of them. A kid at the reins of these things is like putting a blind man at the wheel of a sports car.

The bottom line was that despite being surrounded by people my own age, all of whom were dabbling and experimenting in all kinds of adult vices, I still wasn't tempted to start smoking but I *was* knee-deep in alcohol consumption. We weren't alcoholics but we drank pretty much everyday or whenever it was offered. Nobody said no.

I was also a much fitter man then than I am now and was heavily influenced (as many millions of kids were) by sporting heroes. Many footballers consumed vast amounts of drink without it seeming to affect their performances and goal-scoring skills – George Best was a classic case - unlike today where so much money is invested into sport that drinking excessively is considered bad form. I was to watch 'Boro's football team fluctuate between victories and defeats for many years to come and a few new beer bellies didn't make much difference.

Of course we weren't supposed to drink until we were 18 but nobody gave a damn. As long as we weren't wearing school uniform they took our money in any bar in town so after a year of being a good boy and playing knockout football or five-a-side in the local car parks, a guy a little older than me started to tell me about going out on Friday nights in the town centre. I didn't mix with anybody who did that and had no idea where to start and overcome with shyness, it wasn't fear that stopped me but genuine ignorance. So I went out with this guy one night and hung around with him in a couple of 'Boro bars and within hours bumped into almost half of my ex-schoolmates I hadn't seen for about two years. We were all hovering either just below or just above 18 years old and out of uniform but there we were, drinking like our parents did, not a teacher or Prefect in sight.

So I was now able to spend Friday nights socialising in bars, gradually attracting other young men and girls just like me – uncertain, unsure, a little afraid but overwhelmingly curious about each other. Once we stepped through the door heaving with bodies, smoke and the scent of hops and sugar and familiar noises from the jukebox, we were swept away into the world our parents had enjoyed so much.

Soon I was drinking every Friday and Saturday night with another guy called Bobby a bit like me – shy, curious, clumsy, seeing socialising not only as a chance to learn about adult ways but as a way to meet girls. Bobby lived close to where I lived and with his family, like me. Occasionally during daytimes when he wasn't working – he was working and I wasn't, I was on the dole – we'd listen to each other's music on our stereos. It was with Bobby that I first got steaming drunk on Christmas Eve 1981.

We'd stayed in The Bridge all evening, deliberately wading our way through six pints of cider each. I'd never drunk so much in my young life to that point. Once the drunkenness kicked in – after about four pints – we started to lose the plot. We should have stopped of course but never having been so drunk before we had no idea what we were letting ourselves in for. Added to this was this notion that Christmas was the time to celebrate and in our world that meant drinking lots. The legs went first. We somehow managed to support each other for about half the journey home until neither could walk. I remember him falling down in the middle of the pavement while I managed to stagger home alone, fell through the back door and into the kitchen where the family dog came to greet me and I puked up six pints of cider onto its head. My poor Mam stuck her head around the corner and said something inevitable like: 'Well it had to happen eventually!' cleaned up the puke and threw a blanket over me and I slept on the kitchen floor, waking up on Christmas Day with that most unpleasant experience: the hangover.

The next day I met up with Bobby and he had a go at me for abandoning him but all I could say was that I just wasn't in any frame of mind to care, such was the state of drunkenness we'd both achieved and spent hours doing what we presumed adults did – comparing notes, boasting about it as if it was some rite of passage which in many ways it was and still is.

I was unaware then of how drinking and smoking were an escape from a difficult reality. Literature, movies, art, real situations are all around, all are full of hints and clues as to how a relaxed pleasure turns into a way of life and eventually a destructive addiction, but unless you're experiencing it for yourself you just don't know or can't see how.

It's odd looking back now, emerging from a thirty-year binge, to remember my mind-set back then from the age of 16 to about 21 when I drank regularly. I didn't smoke tobacco or anything else, despite cigarettes being smoked by friends, colleagues and strangers in the street. For those impressionable five years I'd no idea, no understanding and no comprehension of the power of the addiction of tobacco because I didn't smoke. What put me off was that I was still living at home and nobody smoked so being a smoker was always going to be expensive, as I was surviving on dole money alone and impractical. Until I left home I was in a fixed place within the family structure - clothed, sheltered and fed and nowhere within that framework was there any influence of smoking cigarettes. It just wasn't part of my life. If I'd suddenly started smoking my parents would have had an ideal opportunity to put pressure on me to either stop or leave home. Throughout 1983 I'd been slowly saving what little money I had so that when the showdown eventually came I'd have enough to secure a rented room somewhere. And that's exactly what happened in November of that year but if I'd been a smoker I'd have had nothing at all to spare and would have spent it all on fags.

When I finally left home, I moved to sharing a house in Grove Hill not far away, so the transition wasn't difficult. The set-up was similar to the set-up I'd left: a middle-aged woman with two young kids, and her live-in boyfriend. Both had day jobs, responsibilities, no bad addictions and no unpleasant behaviour. I was 'free' from being told to be home at a certain time, turn my music down, not have girls stay overnight, not have to eat when everybody else ate and eat what everybody else ate. Having broken free of my place within the family portrait, I could then redefine my place in the social portrait of a wider world.

For six months or so nothing changed apart from having wilder haircuts and buying and wearing crazier fashions, painting my face like Adam Ant or cutting my hair radically or putting earrings in my nose and ears. I also went vegetarian as a protest against factory farming. But then in the spring of 1984, I fatefully crossed paths with a man who was to have a big influence on my life: a man who died in June 2014 at the age of 52. His name was Jim.

8 – The E Word

Cancer is a group of diseases that involve abnormal increases in the number of cells with the potential to invade or spread to other parts of the body. There are over 100 different known cancers that affect humans. Cancers are often described by the body part that they originated in but for better precision are also classified by the cell the tumor originated from. These types include: carcinoma (common particularly in older adults) breast, prostate, lung, pancreas and colon, sarcoma (cancers in bone, cartilage, fat or nerves), lymphoma and leukaemia (cells that make blood) and Germ Cell (genitourinary and gynecologic cancers often present in the testicle or ovary or bladder, cervix and prostate). There is also Blastoma (cancers derived from embryonic tissue) and cancers in bone and muscles, the brain and the nervous system, the breast, the endocrine system (e.g. thyroid) and on and in the skin (melanoma) and the thoracic and respiratory systems and gastrointestinal (colon, anal). In short, there are over one hundred known cancers that can affect the human body and because cigarette smoke is inhaled into the lungs and spread throughout the body through the blood, all and any part of the human body is therefore susceptible to cancers caused by the chemicals found in used smoke.

But there's another illness that is less talked about but just as effective at shortening life and, particularly, reducing the quality of life and I've seen two examples of it with my own eyes.

Emphysema is a lung condition that causes shortness of breath. In people with emphysema, the air sacs in the lungs (alveoli) are damaged. Over time, the inner walls of the air sacs weaken and rupture, creating larger air spaces instead of many small ones. It is the composition of these smaller air sacs that allows oxygen to be more easily and readily absorbed and then distributed to various parts of the body. The more alveoli our lungs have, the larger the surface area able to absorb oxygen is and the better for the body because it's constantly using oxygen to be as efficient a machine as it can be. But when those little sacs are broken down, for example, they become one sac and this means less oxygen is absorbed into the bloodstream, so though the body may be constantly demanding the same amount of fresh oxygen to keep it functioning as supplied by the little sacs, four fifths less of that supply is now being pumped to it. Plus, when you exhale, the damaged alveoli don't work properly and the old air from the previous breath becomes trapped, leaving no room for the fresh, oxygen-rich air from the next breath to enter.

You can have emphysema for many years without noticing any signs or symptoms. The main symptom of emphysema is shortness of breath, which usually begins gradually. You may start avoiding activities that cause you to be short of breath, so the symptom doesn't become a problem until it starts interfering with daily tasks.

Daily tasks, at first glance, suggest physically demanding jobs like carrying bags or climbing ladders or cleaning windows and in one way those are 'daily tasks'. But once emphysema takes hold 'daily tasks' become even more simplified and, as I have seen with my own eyes, a 'daily task' soon becomes an extremely simple and basic human function. I've seen two examples of people who suffered from advanced emphysema, both women, one over 80 and the other over 50. In both cases they were heavy cigarette smokers from early ages. One was a neighbour of my parents. She wore an oxygen mask and carried a small bottle of it with her everywhere, from the moment she got out of the bed in the morning until the moment she returned to it in the evening, like a deep sea diver floating through an air-free world. She needed the oxygen mask to lift her own upper body weight off the bed and into a sitting position so she could dress herself. She would then use the toilet with the mask on her face and only take it off to wash or shower but could not lift her arms above her head. She lived in a bungalow so she wouldn't have to negotiate stairs. She couldn't climb stairs even if she had wanted to. It didn't mean that with the mask on her face she was suddenly able to live and move around freely. In the cases of both women their emphysema became so advanced that it was one breath = one movement. With the former her emphysema was 'one breath = one sentence or one movement'. With the latter it was worse, it became 'one full lungful of breath = one word' and even those nothing more than whisper. She couldn't even allow herself to lie down on her back in a bed because she wouldn't be able to get back up again and suffocate. She'd to spend every night in an upright sitting position on a chair in her kitchen. In the end she couldn't even talk anymore as it took too much effort to gather in enough breath to operate her voice-box and she had to be fed and cleaned by her devoted son.

The main cause of emphysema is long-term exposure to airborne irritants, including tobacco smoke, marijuana smoke, air pollution or fumes and dust. Occupational hazards can also be included in this category such as workers exposed to exhaust fumes or dust from cotton, wood, coal, stone or petrol. But most are smokers.

9 – The Leader - 1984

When people are seeking a leader, they look for qualities like intelligence, wit, creativity and charisma, but a leader also needs to be motivated and willing to challenge certain ideas and practices. The true psychological profile of a great leader is that he or she is a risk-taker – a similar flaw found in addicts. For me, Jim was a leader *because* he was a risk-taker.

People with risk-taking traits, often found in addicts, can be useful in becoming a leader. For many leaders, it isn't the case that they're able to do well in spite of their addiction; rather, the same chemistry that makes them addicts serve them as leaders. Jim looked like a rock star and behaved like one, despite clearly not being one. True, he played electric bass guitar in some forgotten groups but all small towns have such people – they are often the nearest thing impressionable kids have to real heroes. Their personalities are addictive and this isn't the same as having an addictive personality. People with addictive personalities use addictions to cope in stressful situations ut addiction doesn't cure – it just provides temporary relief from anxiety.

There is some debate about the question of whether an addictive personality really exists at all. Nobody is forced to drink and smoke excessively. The theory of addictive personalities agrees that there are two types of people: risk-takers and risk-averse. Risk-takers enjoy challenges, new experiences and want instant gratification. These people enjoy the excitement of danger and trying new things. On the other hand, risk-averse are those who are by nature cautious. It's the personality traits of individuals that combine to create either risk-taker or risk-averse but it's that same two-way traffic that can also create a mutual dependence.

Arguments against the theory of addictive personality are that by labelling someone with an addictive personality, one may think that there is no way to change the outcome but this label may cause many to believe that there is no way to change this or treat addictions, which, according to many researchers and doctors, is untrue.

For Jim, the cause of death was liver failure aggravated by excessive drinking and drug abuse over a period of about 30 years. I ran alongside him for a parallel period of about the first 10-15 years. I'm still here writing this but he's dead.

Jim looked the part and had a personality to match his appearance: always a black mop-top fluffed up on the top of his head with a fringe either just below his eyebrows or if it got too long he'd sweep it away to each side of his eyes and it'd tumble down to his shoulders. He almost exclusively wore either: a black leather bike jacket or a denim jacket, tight jeans and black boots – winter, spring, summer or autumn, a drink in one hand and cigarette in the other and could be found at just about every party in that small town or every bar.

Specific working class groups populated certain working class pubs and crossing the barriers of acceptance between those groups was considered risky. A young guy could go into a certain pub and get himself beaten to a pulp just because he wore eyeliner. Openly gay men were intimidated and often put in hospital. Longhaired rockers and bikers hung out in certain bars that were known throughout the town and recognised by all social classes as being associated and reserved for longhaired bikers and rockers. It was easy back then to look at long-haired bikers and rockers as 'hippies' of a particular anti-Establishment social order, but in fact there was and is an orthodoxy about them, and intolerance of, for example, homosexuality. Longhaired rockers and bikers aren't supposed to be gay – they're supposed to be macho, fuck chicks, drink a lot, take drugs, fight and ride motorbikes. Rockers and bikers didn't make it a rule to go out and seek 'Trendies' (young guys who would dress and conform to the fashions and tastes of whatever was contemporary and modern) to beat up but Trendies would often go out and seek bikers and Rockers to beat up as it was considered a sign of toughness. Similar tensions occurred in the 60s between Rockers and Mods and again in the 70s between Skinheads and Punks. Rivalry was strong but gender prejudice was not the cause of that conflict. Perhaps these rivalries still exist and have gone underground but with everybody thrown into a big melting pot over the last thirty years it seems more difficult to define who belongs to what. And maybe it doesn't matter and maybe that's the whole point?

10 - What's yours is mine and what's mine is yours

Once I quit smoking for the third and final time, I reinforced my position by becoming more militant. I had never truly been aware of how annoying it was to have to suffer breathing in smoke from tobacco burnt by strangers because I was part of the same addiction. Not only were my olfactory glands immune to it due to being compromised by my own addiction but that even if it hadn't been, I'd not have noticed it purely from a sense of being one of the beneficiaries in the horrible conspiracy. I would be standing on a station platform waiting for a train and somebody standing a few yards away from me would light up and their smoke would drift along on the breeze and invade my nostrils. I'd be walking past an office or building entrance in the street and have to take a slight detour to the edge of the pavement to avoid the hopeless addicts huddled outside. I'd be walking in the street, shopping or just strolling, and I'd have to lower my head or literally not breathe as their smoke wafted around me like a little cloud or I'd be sitting outside a cafe or restaurant trying to enjoy the moment with its fresh air and sunlight and somebody at the next table would be smoking, oblivious to my discomfort. The last time that happened was last August. I was celebrating my 54th birthday with my partner and we'd found a lovely Italian restaurant in Brussels with a charming rear outside garden. We'd chosen the nicest spot in the garden and were the first to arrive there. Then a tourist arrived, took the table next to us and started smoking and I was forced to ask the waiter to move to a more distant but unfortunately less well-placed table. Such is the fragile balance between addicts and ex-addicts, or non-addicts.

I become irritated too when in the company of friends when one of them feels the need to stand up and reach for their paraphernalia and head discreetly for the door, often joined by others who were perhaps more polite and less desperate to maintain their fix – a pleasant conversation in the presence of pleasant people suddenly put on hold while 'It' invades the room and dominates all occupants, not only directly.

About a year after I quit smoking for the last time back in 2012, I returned to a popular local bar and casually asked the barman if I could have one of his cigarettes. He looked at me sternly for a moment and then said: "But you've quit!" and I said that was true but if I asked him for a cigarette, would he give me one? He thought about it for a moment and then said yes he would but first I had to tell him why. I told him that I wanted one and that if he gave me it he wouldn't begrudge me. I asked him if he agreed to those terms and he thought about it for a moment more and said yes. The moment he offered me the box and I slid the single cigarette out from amongst the others, broke it in half in my fingers and crushed what was left by rubbing it between my two palms and dumping the contents into the ashtray. His face turned red and he became angry with me. "Why are you angry?" I asked him. "Because one of those costs about 20 cents and I would have smoked it myself!" he replied. "But you agreed that when it left your box and became my possession that i could do with it what I wanted. I never wanted to smoke it. I only ever planned to destroy it." 'It' was speaking through him, inside him controlling what he thought, felt, said and did. I knew that because if he had been in his normal, right mind he would have understood the logic of my actions immediately but even that supposition is misplaced because if he had been in his normal, right mind he wouldn't have been in possession of a box of cigarettes in the first place.

Which, in a long and convoluted way, brings us to the subject of this chapter: second hand and third hand smoke. It's not enough that smokers poison their bodies but they also have the generosity to inflict it upon people around.

Second hand smoke is when an innocent party is forced to inhale the smoke from burning tobacco or from a smoker's lungs. Third hand smoke is the name given to the minute toxic particles that settle on surfaces surrounding the smoker. You see this in most evidence in or on, for example, the beard of a male smoker, should he have a beard, and is indicated by a coloured streak among the whiskers. But you see it also on the walls, but especially the ceilings, of a smoker's home when the original colour of the paint is replaced by a stain. The lungs of the non-smoker which by definition are never used to process nicotine are much purer and finer (and

thus more fragile and more vulnerable) and so will –
whether we want it or not – still enter into our blood.

Children and babies are, with their spotless immune
systems and purer internal organs, not yet corrupted by
airborne pollutants so therefore more susceptible, not
that smokers especially smoking parents, give a shit.

Critics of this logic – smokers usually or natural cynics -
will say that there is no avoiding the airborne pollutants
of the modern world anyway, or that second hand or
third hand smoke is one of the unfortunate pitfalls of the
art of compromise. They may be right. Nonetheless, non-
smoking wives, partners and children of a smoker have a
one quarter increased\chance of catching the same
diseases.

SIDS: Sudden Infant Death Syndrome, perplexed doctors
and parents for years. Why did perfectly normal babies
die in their cots for no apparent reason? Nobody still
knows for sure but experts now have at least some clues
and the finger of blame points in part to the dangers of
smoking when pregnant and being exposed to second

and third hand smoke when pregnant, as well as stillborn births, low weight births and delivery difficulties.

Over the years in which I smoked, I'd often end up in relationships with women who also smoked. Only once or twice did I have relationships with women who didn't smoke but who never objected to the fact that I did and so I inflicted my foul-smelling breath on them when we kissed or I infected the places where they lived. I was self-deluding enough to think to myself "Oh yes we've got lots of things in common – we like the same music, the same food, the same movies and we both smoke!"

In the last five years I've been with one woman for about four of those years and though I didn't 'select' her as my partner because she smoked or not, I was already out of that world by the time we met. When I met my current partner only about a month after I quit, it was her bright, white smile and blue eyes that attracted me most and for the first time in many years I realised what a wonderful world I'd been missing out on for my own want of courage.

11 – Poverty in youth - 1985

Also in Middlesbrough at that time was a 'chapter', of
Hell's Angels – a loose association of so-called lawless
bikers who survived on the outskirts of society through
their own choice and defined tough, fairly macho rules
by which to live. Their mode of transport was the
motorcycle and it was rarely a brightly-coloured
Japanese bike but almost exclusively a classic road-bike
like a Triumph, a BSA or a Harley Davidson. Many of
their bikes were 'souped-up', customised to move faster
than they appeared or have elongated chassis, wider
handlebars or seats for passengers. Their mode of
fashion was basic – black leather, denim, tattoos,
sunglasses and, lots of drinking, sex, rock music and of
course, inevitably, drugs. From a young age I remember
seeing these guys riding around town, silencers removed
in order to be as loud and as intimidating as possible.
The leader was a big guy with a long beard and on his
old-style crash helmet he'd fastened a fox fur down the
middle. Some even sported jackets with Nazi insignia,
which in a still-patriotic, post-war Great Britain was
considered very shocking. They didn't call themselves

by normal Christian names but by nicknames instead like 'Dirtbox' (for his lack of hygiene), 'Killer' (for talking himself out of tricky situations rather than through violence) and 'Ragman' (for want of a better wardrobe). As chance would have it my primary school was in Rosecroft Avenue and on one corner was an old, almost-derelict detached building where the Hell's Angels lived. The building had windows but they'd painted them black so there was no way of anybody on the outside seeing inside and vice versa. By the time the 80's came around this building had become something of a local legend, taking the name 'The Dive'. I never went inside. These guys just weren't my type of people. In fact, they scared the shit out of me, which I think was their intention. But day-time or night-time I'd often pass the place and hear throbbing music pumping through the walls or see bikes parked up outside.

No one was ever sure how he achieved it but Jim managed on a number of occasions to get invited inside and for this badge of courage he shot up in the estimation of those who knew him. Again it was probably those charismatic, risk-taking qualities. Jim went there because he thought he might find drugs, or the rumours were they knew people where drugs could be found and bought, as finding drugs in 'Boro at that time was probably difficult. I say probably because I was standing on the threshold of the entrance door to that world at that time so I really wouldn't have known if they were difficult to find or not, but I can vouch for this by recalling some of the twists and turns I had to take to get drugs later on. For Jim the acquisition and consumption of drugs was a vital step in the journey of the young rebel.

But I'd be wrong to say that that one person was the reason I got into smoking dope and then name that person as Jim as that would be besmirching his name and sounding as if I wasn't accepting responsibility. Drug culture at that time was associated with the hippy or punk lifestyle and representatives of that lifestyle were mostly found in music and in literature. To young, bored, small town kids, replicating the vices of the rich and famous was one way of trying to glimpse a lifestyle beyond us in the hope we might share the same thrills and sensations. The fact that some of them had overdoses and died didn't daunt us in the slightest. Death from drugs was the same as any other introduction to the Reaper: luck, circumstance or fate though obviously none of us wanted to dabble in drugs and die, so I guess we kind of crossed ourselves and secretly said: 'With a bit of luck I can make it out of the other end of this experience in one piece'.

Youth culture had found its voice first in the 1950s with working class teddy boys and rockers. This had then given way to the hippy 1960s when music and politics got mixed together and then in the 1970s came a backlash of heavy rock, stadium rock and disco escapism. In the mid to late 1970s there was yet another backlash in the form of punk rock and acted as a catharsis for other sub-cultures like Ska, New Wave and alternative music. From this synth-pop crossed over into popular culture as the Microchip began to makes its presence felt on the dance floor as well as in the workplace and the home. And of course around each of these new sub-cultures new worlds of fashion spun off in all directions, sometimes colliding, intermingling and creating complex sub-cultures. Anti-war and anti-imperialism had grown out of 1960s peace movements like CND. Anti-Imperialism was largely directed against the two Superpowers. At Greenham Common in Hertfordshire, the American military wanted to install nuclear strike weapons and mass passive revolt eventually managed to curtail that. It was a dangerous and exciting time to be young and alive and the blind argument seemed naïve and blind today but we'd often say: 'Well we might all be dead tomorrow so who gives a fuck?' though different people had different version of what 'fun' constituted. For my friends and I 'fun' was drugs and drink consumed together and in excess to render us so oblivious to reality that we were cushioned against it, for a little while anyway. Having left home and starting to hang around with people my own age in a place where we could dream, fantasise and experiment as young adults, adrift with real money to spend, products of a modern capitalism consumer society seeking short-term thrills, we could do no better than get fucked up.

Somehow or other I ended up round at Jim's flat. At that time Jim was involved in a couple of local music groups as a guitarist though never anything fixed or regular – if he was free and had time to learn the songs, he'd play.

He shared the flat with his flatmate Harry; neither had jobs though Harry did occasionally work as a roadie for local bands. Nobody I knew had a job and I knew a lot of people. We were all either unemployed or students and within this tight network we managed to hustle one another to survive, occasionally turning up some cash from somewhere but more than likely blowing it on fast food, drink and drugs. Quite how we made it through those days is a bit of a mystery to me today but I'm speaking now from a middle aged standpoint, from a routine where I'm used to having fixed meals at fixed times and where the alcohol intake is limited. Back then we had so little money to spare that doing something wise with it - like spending it on heating bills, rent and food - was just the last thing to do. Heating was generally paid for by buying tokens so we'd at least be guaranteed some heat for a certain number of days but when the token ran out, we froze or went to bed to stay warm. We tried to pay the rent but the idea of a monthly bank transaction that automatically took the rent from our accounts was unknown back then and the landlord would often come round to the door – if we didn't have the rent we'd not answer. As for food, we lived on the minimum of cheap foods from cheap supermarkets but so we didn't end up living in some sort of monotonous wasteland, we'd have blow-outs usually on the day the dole cheque arrived - a trip to the local curry house or chip shop or kebab shop but what remained – if anything – went on drink, sometimes in cans and bottles from the off-licence but more often than not in bars and pubs because in a bar or pub you had a combination of elements that made life bearable: heat, social life and alcohol. Those of us lucky enough to have parents living close by occasionally got to go home and get stocked up with food or money, as I did, so it was never the end of the world.

Shopping for new clothes was impossible on the budgets we had so we either got hand-me-down's from the family or bought cheap in charity shops. The only thing we never stinted on in our youth culture was footwear – trainers, shoes or boots we always made an effort to pay full whack for those and once we had them we wore them until they literally dropped off, in summer, autumn, spring and winter especially.

We shoplifted food when we were desperate – which was often. The local all-night garage on the A167 was easy to steal from but we were unlikely to find wholesome foodstuffs in an all night garage and often ended up stealing chocolate because as newcomers to dope we'd experience what's commonly known as the 'munchies'. The chemical compound in dope (cannabis resin or hashish) robs the blood of sugar so the body has a sudden urge to compensate by hungrily consuming more and that was easily available in chocolate, another reason we spent so much time stealing as well as eating chocolate bars!

For the two years I lived in Middlesbrough independently I smoked hash regularly, but never grass or marijuana. Grass was seen as a luxury for the wealthy or people in hot countries. Everybody I knew involved in drugs smoked hashish. To us in North East England it usually came through the seaports like Sunderland, Newcastle or Blyth. Sailors looking to boost their incomes would buy thick wedges of hashish, fill up a hold-all in some foreign port and when they got it to England either sell it off to dealer at twice the price they paid or process it themselves. This meant cutting up the slabs into recognised 'street' weights. The most common weight for us and most people I knew was a sixteenth of an ounce or an eighth of an ounce, going by their street tags 'an eighth' (or a Henry, Henry VIII) or 'a sixteenth'. On dole wages most of us bought – when we could – a sixteenth, which was about enough for half a dozen joints. An eighth was considered a luxury, as it would cost about a quarter of our dole money.

Dole money back then was paid once a fortnight and in the form of a green giro cheque. We'd sign on for the money by going to a specific building at a specific time, queuing and signing a card and then two days later the cheque would usually arrive at our homes in the post. We'd take the cheque to our nearest post office with some form of ID and they'd exchange it for cash. It was a struggle to get out of the post office without spending anything on fags or chocolate. From that moment the money would be burning a hole in our pockets and, having usually starved or lived like monks for the last couple of days before signing on. It'd only be a matter of hours before half was gone and it'd start all over again the same cycle of debt.

Thanks to a mutual network of friends in similar positions though, we'd be able to borrow small amounts, as we'd have alternate signing on weeks. One week I'd have some cash and my mate wouldn't, so I'd lend him a couple of pounds to help him get through that week and then the next week I'd have nothing left but he'd receive his dole, so he'd lend me a couple of pounds to help me get through. It was by this kind of leapfrogging that we managed to keep going but other than this pitiful income we soon began to understand how tobacco, dope and booze fended off the reality of crushing poverty. At the same time, if we hadn't smoked or drunk, we might have just about had enough to get by on the dole. It depends largely how you look at State Welfare; in some countries people on welfare are classed as scroungers, deficient or lacking something cerebrally to allow themselves to lose their jobs, be made redundant or fired.

It meant shopping in stores where no frills (such as extravagant packaging or industrially produced food) governed the weekly budget. It meant not buying good, vitamin-packed, quality food but cheap fatty food to keep hunger at bay. I used to buy Fine Fare's own brand of fish fingers in a plain white box with a dozen fish fingers made up of the fins, eyes, the tail and every part of the fish except the fillets. For many of us, our only vice was sugar as it offered us something cheap and sweet every time we drank a cup of tea or coffee and it took me years to figure out that I wasn't really enjoying the taste of coffee or milk but using coffee and milk as an excuse to deliver sugar into my system.

From 1983 to 1985 I lived away from the family home and somehow managed to stay alive whilst subsisting on the margins. At any time I could have put aside my personal prejudices against working and within a month be making money and paying taxes like everyone else. But it was mostly terror for me at that age, knowing how to manage the vacuum of purpose once the destiny of the Welder had been stolen. I chose to be an 'angry young man' who hated the rich or anyone who pronounced glass like arse or going as 'gonna'. It was a defence against the humiliation forced on me by the nameless, faceless bastards who drove up to the shipyard offices in brand new cars and wearing suits, shirts and ties. I was robbed of my identity of Welder with a capital W but knew I had to hold my head high. We all did. I'd drifted into a chip-on-my-shoulder territory at the age of 15 because I really didn't have a clue what was going on in the adult world, after leaving school with no qualifications. I wasn't remotely politicised, self-aware or self-disciplined. I'd just fallen into the working life routine like my father and his before him stretching back a couple of centuries. For a little over two years I'd got a weekly wage and lived at home, paid some 'board' and been fed and clothed. Suddenly, in 1982, I was redundant. So for another two years I stayed living at home and signing on and paying board. In November 1983, no longer able to knuckle under to the house rules, I was out in the cold world on my own with no job, no money and only a little parental support ('You can come back and have a nice hot meal once a week if you like?').

I soon noticed that tobacco kept hunger at bay so the wisest thing to do seemed to me to be to hang out with other people in the same boat – living alone or sharing, but certainly not with their families and signing on. We were all unemployed. Most of our fathers had been employed in the shipyards or factories too. They were suddenly wiped out under Thatcher.

In October 1984 I'd left the attic flat I was living in after first leaving home to share a flat with a painter called Chris. Chris was ten years older than me.

Through 1984 into 1985 I struggled on, drinking when I could afford it and smoking other people's dope when it was offered, despite having barely two pennies to rub together. I got by through buying and selling records or fanzines when the dole money dried up. I've always loved pop and rock music from the last 60 years. In my youth I kept in contact with music by buying cheap records whenever I could, often at knockdown prices in reduced to clear bargain bins or second-hand record shops but ultimately I recognised it as a form of throwaway culture in the sense that for me music was a bit like a book – an experience. Keeping hold of all the books I read and all the records I bought and piling them up on shelves wasn't to impress my friends with how intellectual I thought myself. Books, like songs and music, were to me 'momentary' and some books and records endured or appealed more or less depending on needs or tastes, so why hang onto something I don't really care about or has served its purpose? It was by this form of cheap recycling that I kept going through 1984 – the start of the Miner's Strike in the UK.

12 - Smile!

I can't say I particularly felt the effects of smoking on my teeth as a prime motivator to stop in the first place. I'd forever had to visit the dentists every few months for a filling or a clean or, the most dreaded of all, an extraction. The teeth weren't the only things to suffer over the years of abuse, the gums did badly too. Not only did they change colour but also shrank and thus made the security of my remaining teeth less certain. The area of gum that held them in place receded and tiny gaps began to appear, especially lower down the sides of the teeth. I've noticed how people who have healthy teeth don't have these gaps between theirs and not only are their smiles invariably blindingly white – an effect I've never been able to have on the world – but also had a really solid and sturdy look about them.

As a smoker I had never really understood or known how it tasted or felt to kiss another smoker because we'd both had had the same tastes and odours in our mouths. It was only after I quit that, once or twice when I'd met another smoker and had some sort of intimate contact with them, was I on the receiving end! And it was VILE! What really put me off kissing smokers wasn't so much the taste and odour but the fact that 'It' was somehow mocking me through the mouth of another human being. The smoker kissing me was as blissfully unaware of how obnoxious they were being as I had been when I was a smoker kissing non-smokers yet It was somehow still present in that intimate exchange and must have been rubbing the old hands together in glee and gurgling with delight like a kid on Christmas Day to realise that it was still capable of penetrating my defences in such a sly way!

I quit smoking and restarted again at least three significant times in my adult life. One such occasion was back in 2001 when I was living with my now ex-wife Sarah who also had a seven year old son, Louis. I'd drifted into a relationship with Sarah, a non-smoker, but back in those days smoking was still 'accepted', which is to say unopposed indoors or in the daily life. Smokers weren't yet treated as outcasts or banished from indoor spaces to the doorstep or the garden. It was, in fact, such an accepted and normal part of my every-waking-moment existence that I never thought about how Sarah and Louis might feel about it or whether or not they liked it. It was bold, rude and presumptive. An ashtray was found and kept permanently nearby or I carried it around the house we shared from room to room. So of course quite soon into this relationship with Sarah I realised that I wasn't setting much of an example to little Louis. If ever an addict needed an excuse to stop, that was it.

My gums, more than my teeth, were the real victims of my smoking. They frequently bled when I brushed. But the bad news is that even for a period of up to FIVE YEARS after quitting, there is still the risk of increased decay and tooth loss as the mouth recovers from the abuse it has been receiving.

The second time I made a serious effort to stop my addiction was around 2002. I'd maintained my discipline for over a year because of the role I was playing in influencing positive behaviour in my young and impressionable stepson, but at some point my ex-wife and I asked for a small envelope of marijuana from a friend and we then took it away with us for a few days 'fun'. Anxious to avoid mixing the weed with tobacco so as not to restart smoking again – a problem I had and yet not one shared by my ex-wife who though she smoked joints with me was never tempted to restart smoking tobacco – I tried rolling pure joints, that is: no tobacco at all. It was about then that I learned from experience that importing the effects of burnt marijuana into the bloodstream in order to temporarily influence consciousness was almost impossible without tobacco or a small pipe. Tobacco was the main source of heat and as the joint was smoked, the smoker sucked oxygen through the burning tip and fresh burnt smoke moved directly into the lungs. Without tobacco, the marijuana burnt for only a second, ignited by the heat of the catalyser before going out again. I could feel almost straight away that urge to get 'It' back into my life again, to associate the action with the result and the familiarity of the old habit returning. So like a fool I bought some rolling tobacco to mix with our marijuana and though we certainly enjoyed the marijuana itself as long as it lasted, I knew that I had deliberately and voluntarily broken my own rule. From that moment on my smoking became secretive in order to try to maintain the lie to my stepson that my discipline was being maintained. It was back. To hide It from my stepson, not only did I begin a regime of not smoking when he was around but also in disguising my bad breath by eating copious numbers of sugar-filled mints to try to camouflage the smell of smoke so in effect my gums and teeth were now being abused and attacked by smoke and my teeth by excessively sweet mints.

I suffered from 'smoker's palate' and 'coated tongue'. The first is where the roof of my mouth turned white and, I noticed after excessive smoking bouts, very dry with tiny spots which I now know were blocked saliva ducts. Cigarette smoke decreases the production of saliva by blocking the ducts that produce it. This in turn leads to a build up of plaque or calculus as the experts call it. Calculus is the harder form of plaque and is most evident around the teeth of people who do not floss regularly.

'Coated tongue' is even more disgusting: a microscopically thin layer of food particles and collected bacteria from burnt carcinogens on the surface of the tongue, again blocking saliva ducts which influence ability to taste. The dryness in the mouth caused by tobacco smoking is simply to do with the high temperatures during the process to which the interior is subjected. To counter this, the recipient usually drinks more when out socialising and this inevitably means more alcohol to compensate for the dryness. But alcohol attacks the Central Nervous System's ability to regulate itself at reasonable levels and thus to make reasonable decisions, but once that discipline is broken the two, alcohol and cigarette smoking, connect and cancel each other in equal measures in a fast spiral down. A combination of tobacco smoking and alcohol intake increase the risk of oral cancer by between 75-90%. The mouth itself – just as with certain other organs in the human body which are enclosed spaces such as the lungs or intestines - are protected by something called the 'epithelium', which, according to most dictionaries, is a very fine layer of tissue film designed to protect the aforesaid. It acts kind of like a raincoat acts to protect the person that wears it from the dampness of rain. Alcohol simply makes the epithelium more porous. If, therefore, smokers drink more to compensate for the dryness in their mouths of smoking, they reduce the effectiveness of the mouth to protect from diseases and from cancers.

The worst case scenario from oral cancer brought on by excessive smoking and alcohol intake I ever heard of was the case of the actor Jack Wild, perhaps best known for his role as the Artful Dodger in the 1969 musical film 'Oliver!' His consumption of tobacco and alcohol caused him to have his entire tongue removed.

Crowns and bridges are also positive additions to dental improvements but all the hard work and expense that they take to fit and install is lost when fitted into the mouth of a smoker. In 2009 I spent €2000 and many hours on the installation of a bridge to conceal and cover a very ugly upper left line of old, broken teeth. A year later when I moved to Paris I started smoking again. Idiot.

13 – Philosophies of the 80's

The Miner's Strike was only one of a multitude of trans-global events and realities that young people lived with in those days. The imminent threat of nuclear war between America and Russia was another. At some point in my youth I'd been informed of the existence of weapons that could wipe out humanity and that fear was reflected in the tensions that existed between the political East and West – the Cold War. Naturally it scared and depressed me, as it scares and depresses most people, especially on that bizarre day when, usually as a child, an adult informs you of the situation. It's at that point (or just after) you find yourself thinking: 'Well what's the bloody point in going on if we're all going to end up in ashes?' Not to say that this is a reason to become a drunk or a drug addict but tension is there and it's never going away.

I'd passed through the experience of The Falkland's Conflict between Britain and Argentina in 1982 and around the time the news was breaking and me and all my friends were thinking: 'The end is nigh!' but look at the state of the world today: over-population, unclean air, dwindling resources, global-warming, terrorism everywhere, and it's hard to envisage a safe future, so for a large number of people these problems-without-solutions become an instigator of a general sense of helplessness. Long story short: apart from recycling vinyl records, occasional odd jobs washing cars or shoplifting, I scraped through that year by the skin of my teeth and if I stumbled onto drugs (I was well established as a drinker by then) it was only a way in which to suspend the reality of my situation and make it bearable.

At some point I moved from being just an imbiber of other people's drugs to buying my own and thus being able to choose when and where and with whom I wanted to be stoned. That was a big fundamental 'next step' in the process. Tasting something offered by friends means that when you leave that situation the effects wear off and you return to your natural state and in that natural state you can get on with your life and get things done. But when you consciously go out and buy an eighth of an ounce of hash (which took up about half my dole money for a fortnight) it meant that I had the ability to smoke non-stop for a few days. The price you pay for being off your head is time. You waste and fritter it with such casualness it's frightening.

The influence of counter-culture in the form of rock and roll had an enormous influence on drug taking amongst 'ordinary' people. Drugs are seen as a passport to a glamorous world that our heroes inhabit, on our music stereos, onstage in front of thousands or on our screens. Rock and roll legends sometimes die under the influence of drugs and are worshipped as if dying in a stupor of breathlessness or vomit is heroic. Destiny for them isn't getting old, wrinkled and falling to pieces but leaving the world young and remembered as such forever, though for the most part their talent is snuffed out and they'll produce nothing more.

I learnt to roll spliffs or joints. It was Jim who taught me of course. I've since learned that people roll joints in a variety of ways. This meant familiarising myself – in England anyway – with the Rizla: thin, feather-light wafers of paper used to encase loose tobacco to be smoked as the ubiquitous 'Rollie'. At first touch I was amazed at how fragile these papers – in common parlance referred to as skins – actually are. Dextrous fingers and thumbs are often used to handling objects with some weight, shape and form but I was used to handling heavy working tools with a light touch. The lightness of a skin was something different. Jim made his joints using four skins and I copied, my first few attempts being useless, but I soon got the hang of it and then reduced it to three and now two.

One of the disadvantages to smoking hashish is its density; it is in fact compacted marijuana plant 'heads' (un-pollinated flowers). Marijuana plant heads can be dried out and then smoked by crumbling the green leaves and sticky flowers into the tobacco, but hashish is a more compact version of this. Hashish is invariably brown but as it comes from plants from all over the world with climates hot enough to support their growth, not only are the plants a multitude of different strengths but their colours are too. Almost all dope starts its life with strength in it but the longer it rests in its compacted state or the more it's exposed to air, the less potent it becomes and, unless one had a good contact back in those days, by the time it trickled down to small-time end-users like us it was a fraction of its quality, though that didn't stop it being five or six times more expensive from source. As for 'quality control' – forget it. If you score (a slang word for buy) dope and its doesn't do anything to your head then it's safe to say you've been ripped-off but the only way you can complain is by moaning and the only person you can moan to is the person you bought it off but there isn't going to be any refund or exchange so good luck with that one.

14 - A good hockle

'Hockle' is one of many verbs used to discern the noise a person makes in their throat when trying to manoeuvre an obstructive mass of mucus into a position where they can eject it from the body by spitting. There are other more popular nouns such as snot, bogies and phlegm but neither of these lends themselves so easily to noun and verb. A hockle is something you do or have but once out of the body can take any other number of labels. The hockle particularly came into fashion once the chewing of tobacco became popular and 'spittoons' – bowl-shaped metal objects - were scattered around the floors of many drinking bars so people could spit out the tobacco juice. However, the emptying and cleaning of such receptacles must have required a particular mark of courage. The outdoors and especially green spaces of today are still considered by the vast majority of men (hockling seems to be reserved to male culture) as open ground for clearing the lungs as long as what they leave behind isn't too excessive or revolting or likely to come into contact with anyone or anything else. Having said that, anyone with even half a brain knows that not to negotiate the streets and walkways of today's world by looking down as much as one looks up is an invitation for a variety of excreted and dumped human or animal waste to end up on one's shoes.

Phlegm (mucus), to give it its more official name, is a sticky fluid that plays an important role in the respiratory system: it traps dust, bacteria and viruses that get slowly propelled towards the throat by the cilia: the tiny hairs that line the airways. This is quite normal – the respiratory system depends on mucus to lubricate the airways but excess phlegm production isn't normal and can have different causes like over-exposure to irritants, pollutants or allergy-causing substances. For example, having a wet cough or chest congestion is a sign of too much phlegm. When it's excessive or thick, the cilia can become overworked, prompting the cough reflex to clear the excess.

Overproduction of mucus can be caused by allergens such as dust mites or pollen. The body boosts mucus production as it tries to fight the infection or smoke, mould, car exhaust or certain chemicals. Smokers lungs are exposed to twice the levels of airborne particles compared to non-smokers so more mucus is produced in the respiratory system of smokers as the lungs and airways work overtime trying to clear these pollutants. Constant coughing and long-term smoking can also directly provoke mucus production, as can Lung Disease. COPD refers to a group of diseases and emphysema and bronchitis are among them.

15 – Through the Gateway – 1984 & 1985

At some point in early 1985 I entered into a new realm: I bought my own dope, tobacco and skins and would waste hours or days at a time with Chris or others who would pop round our flat and we'd smoke and smoke until it was gone. Chris would paint, but just as often we'd talk crap, giggle a lot and eat stolen chocolate.

I think it's probably also safe to say that when you smoke tobacco you also end up smoking dope, or at least try it. To smoke dope you really need to smoke tobacco as well. The two things, for me, went hand in hand. When the dope ran out I continued smoking the tobacco under the misguided belief that I'd still be kind of getting something off the experience, but it was bollocks of course, it wasn't doing anything except ruining my health and taking cash from my pockets.

Living with Chris, both of us totally broke, we ended up regularly shoplifting at the local late-night garages, sweet shops or supermarkets. Even a blind man can see how so many anti-social actions are connected - lack of education and opportunities - lack of potential – poverty - escape from poverty - drugs and drinking - petty thieving - crime – poor judgement and so on. You don't have to be a genius to work it out. The one thing that stopped me sliding inexorably to a far worse lifestyle than I ended up flirting with was a love of art and culture. That was what saved me from oblivion back in those early days – art and culture.

Having said that, 21st June 1984 seemed to many to be a significant date, not only the year George Orwell predicted (in his book of the same name) that we'd be living under a harsh dictatorship (and there were glimmers) but also the longest day of the year and alternative 'religions' and society's 'outcasts' celebrated the Summer Solstice by flocking en masse to places like Stonehenge. So did I.

I hitchhiked there and over the course of the day set up tent near the soundstage. Stonehenge had been a regular visiting spot for hippies since the 60's and attending this freeform celebration seemed like a stab at liberty. In 1985 Thatcher was top dog. Having 'beaten the Argies' and then Scargill and his Miner's Strike that ended in March 1985, Stonehenge Festival was also banned. Although I didn't know it at the time, 1984 was the last big free event. I didn't partake in any of the multitude of drugs on offer back then though because although I was curious I was still afraid of what would happen. But drugs were there at the Festival and the numerous film crews, journalists and plain-clothes policemen who visited the sight would have seen flagrant law breaking governing controlled substances.

On a 21st birthday it's traditional in Britain to see it as a bridge between youth and adulthood, though some would argue those boundaries have become blurred. Nonetheless, the UK has always celebrated being 21 and it was no different when I hit 21 – my parents gave me £100 to do with as I liked. If I'd been a sensible boy I'd have used it to buy some new clothes or stocked up my pantry but I lived in poverty so when somebody suddenly put £100 into my hand (a 2018 equivalent is just under £400) when I'd been scraping by at £17.50 a week dole, it's hard to be sensible, especially when you've discovered drug culture.

For Chris, I think drug taking was a key to a 'door of perception' (I know I'm quoting Aldous Huxley here and making strong references to The Doors and Jim Morrison but let's face it - he got there long before me). Chris was a painter who worked in a Neo or Post-Impressionist style: faces, lines and forms were blurred and never clear or defined. The kitchen of the flat we shared was full of FOR SALE signs he'd stolen from gardens to prime and use as 'canvasses' to paint on. There was an easel too, near the kitchen sink, and he'd spend hours happily smoking rolled-up cigarettes, drinking coffee or beer, gradually getting more and more fucked up but painting, always painting, the sedating influence gradually creeping along from his brain to his fingertips that held the brushes, reflecting more and more the blurred visions, as if reflecting his own.

16 - The Junkie and his Works

You might see pictures of a heroin addict with their punctured arms, dirty fingernails and smelly clothes and lolling heads and think to yourself 'That's not me and will never be!' and in one way that's true – it isn't you. You're probably not a heroin junkie. What would kill a heroin junkie is not what would kill a tobacco junkie. A heroin junkie might die from the fact the heroin they are injecting is too pure or the object of injection – the syringe – is infected. There are no cases of people dying from too-pure forms of tobacco but though tobacco smokers have no blood contact with another person though the filters of shared cigarettes and joints, saliva contact is still made.

But in another way it IS you. Because what the smoker and the junkie have in common – apart from the fact that it's usually the case that both parties are trapped in a cycle of self-destruction – is that you both have certain objects about your persons (or in your home) via which you are able to deliver your drugs to your bodies. For the junkie this is usually a small teaspoon on which to heat the heroin until it liquefies enough to be able to be transferred to their syringe and then something to tie around the arm as a tourniquet to restrict blood flow.

The tobacco smoker will have either a standard pipe or a box of ready-made cigarettes or a packet of rolling tobacco, often with the rolling papers inside the pouch, sometimes with small pieces of card to use as filters and something combustible. But for all intents and purposes, the tobacco smoker might just as well also have a syringe handy in which to inject small amounts of liquid nicotine into their veins, as smoke it via a cigarette. In both cases the blood is the main transporter of the drug to their body.

17 – London Arrival - 1986

Like a red flag to a bull, what had been sporadic in Middlesbrough where I'd never even had a regular dealer, became methodical in London. London was bursting to the seams with stress and corruption on just about every conceivable level. Jim moved down from 'Boro six months later. I went to see him in a squat near Kennington Oval. He was living with tight-knit emigrants from all over the UK and Ireland, some of whom were injecting heroin and sharing needles.

I ended up living in a shared house in Hackney run by a housing association, which meant each person got a room but had to share the kitchen, bathroom or communal areas like living rooms. Living in such close-quarter conditions with a wide variety of people from all walks of life meant drugs were rife. There was always somebody (most houses had between four of six tenants) in a house that smoked and always somebody who smoked dope or knew where to get it.

I started subsidising my life by working in bars and pubs. The pubs were often populated with dealers who used them as kind of un-official shops, not to mention the nightclubs where they were sanctioned by owners and organisers in return for a cut. My new 'mates' had close contact with drug dealers.

Within days of moving to London I was smoking Benson and Hedges. I never smoked them in Middlesbrough, I couldn't afford to. I could say now that I don't know why I was smoking them but in truth I do – it's because I was a sucker for the marketing and wrapping and because I had £700 life savings in my bank account. I'd never, after 20 years of life, been responsible for such a large amount. The cigarette box was covered in gold-coloured wrapping and the combination of that and the name went hand-in-hand. I could kind of half-convince myself that I was prestigious because I smoked them. They were certainly stronger than Silk Cut or Embassy Extra Mild. To smoke Benson & Hedges singled me out as 'hardcore' which in terms of prestige meant that I was a risk-taker. Even as I write this I see now how ridiculous it all sounds, but back then I couldn't; I didn't have thirty years experience to draw on. I'd always prided myself that I'd never be a sucker for advertising and I was one-step ahead of the other suckers, but it was a complete lie. I later passed over to Winston for the same stupid reason - because I thought they were unique and therefore that made me more unique. I smoked Marlboro and even Camel too – it was all in the packaging really, this insane idea that being seen in a bar holding a particular box would attract other people to me, whether male or female.

Rolling a cigarette from a wafer-thin skin and a small pinch of tobacco is an acquired talent, especially when you're in a hurry or it's windy or rainy. Nonetheless, hardened smokers convince themselves that they have some kind of amazing skill. Rolled cigarettes are shorter than manufactured cigarettes and burn down more slowly, often needing a light to rekindle them as not drawing on the tip for any length of time means that it extinguishes itself. Making rollies when driving a car is fraught with danger - do you have time to fill a skin with enough tobacco, get it rolled into a tight-ish tube, into your mouth and lit *before* the lights change from red to green? Have a fatal accident at this point and you *can* honestly say 'Smoking Kills'.

Largely for the sake of cost and partially because of the smell, I switched to rolling tobacco but these were the only two reasons. Pound for pound it was no cheaper and no less of a drain on my pocket. Measuring an addiction financially is another way of course of finding an argument against it but at the end of the day, it's probably the weakest of all the motives. Look at the cost of cigarettes today in the UK – around £8 for 20 and yet people are still smoking and the black market is thriving. In the late 1980s I bought boxes of ten and they cost me about 80p. I'd budget my life at £1.50 a day – 80p for ten fags, 30p for a pint of milk and 40p for a tin of beans – all I needed to keep starvation from the door.

Once I'd established a way of maintaining my addiction, I was then free to roam the underground world of London, the illegal and shady nervous system that lurks just beneath the veneer of respectability, to plunder the drugs on offer.

All cigarette smokers leave stubs so I soon turned to what is one of the most degrading things an addict can do: roll up the used stubs from the ashtrays into my own cigarette papers and smoke them. I remember going to parties in the 80's emptying full ashtrays into plastic bags and taking them home, rolling out left-over tobacco from other people's cigarettes and rollies. Up until two years ago, just before I quit, I was doing the same thing with joints. In the tip of almost every joint there's a crumb or two of dope so if you crumble the remains onto another skin you can just about scrape together one more spliff from the remnants. It was a revolting habit I carried with me up until almost the last minute, even though I told myself to stop because there was no dignity in it. But there was never any dignity anyway.

Also sharing the same house was my friend Michael. Michael (like Chris in Middlesbrough) had studied as a Fine Artist but slipped on the banana skin also known as a friend of a friend who one day innocently asks: 'Anybody want to try some heroin?' So began Michael's long nightmare, a personal hell of heroin addiction. He'd injected on a daily basis, destroying veins in his arms, legs and belly, even injecting into his dick occasionally.

I met Michael shortly after I'd moved into the house in Hackney. He'd managed to kick his habit and was still going through his methadone programme – the prescribed substitute favoured by the medical profession to wean addicts off heroin without over-harsh withdrawal. As part of the routine, Michael had to be vetted by the other residents of the house, but on the day he turned up I was the only one who bothered to make the effort to meet him and we got on, so I ok'd him to move in and he did. He wore his methadone programme on his lapel and didn't try to hide it, trading his official prescription with junkies that often hung around the door of RELEASE, the charitable body set up to help drug addicts in London. Michael smoked heavily – tobacco and dope – and drank Carlsberg Special Brew as he found being zonked out most of the time was the only way he could live with the withdrawal. A number of times he tried to find the words to describe the 'heavenly' feelings he'd endured when he'd injected heroin. I never once recall him telling me the 'high' wasn't amazing. But the price was a gradual poisoning, reduced efficiency of the internal organs, drying of skin, eczema, rotten teeth, body sores and so on.

So, yes, there was a kind of a habit for me too in that I inadvertently (or unwittingly) befriended and was mentored and strongly influenced by three men older than me by about ten years – Chris, Pete and Michael - who'd all risen in their fields and shown latent talent but taken bad gambles and paid heavy prices. It wasn't that I admired them because they had kamikaze tendencies or a predilection for risk-taking but that they were all intelligent, sensitive and creative men who'd clung on to art as a panacea or *raison d'etre*. Indeed, in two of the cases it was that natural creativity that had pulled them back from death's door. I felt that in their wisdom there was some loose guidance for my own life choices, like art and culture, but not drug choices. Somebody else said it better than me but it's not about great or good or rich or poor – it's all about the passion you have for your art. The fact that each of these three men wrestled with their own inner demons wasn't so much that I made the choice to be influenced because of those addictions of but in spite of them.

But towards the late 1980s and early 1990s, Mafia-controlled drugs production multiplied as demand skyrocketed. Drug culture probably increased (I'm hedging my bets because I've no hard evidence other than what I witnessed myself) because of popular culture. Music was a large conduit. Some British groups like Happy Mondays and the Stone Roses started openly talking about drug consumption in their songs – a blatant hit record in 1992 was 'Ebenezer Goode' by the Shamen which had the daring chorus line 'E's are good, E's are good, 'e's Ebenezer Goode' and used a Victorian Scrooge-like character to describe the effects of Ecstasy. The music scene changed almost overnight and dance and trance music (coming out of the earlier house music and rap scenes) with high-energy tunes with repetitive beats without names of artists or names emerged. These tracks went on with slight variations on the same theme, music designed to support the mental and physical effects provoked by Ecstasy. Ecstasy threw aside inhibitions between strangers and suddenly nobody was

ashamed of being a crap dancer. It was false of course –
it was simply what the drug was making us think, rather
than what we were really thinking but that was the key to
unlocking so many fears.

By 1989 the Tories and Thatcher had been in power for
almost ten years and had won election after election and
I think a kind of inevitable: 'What's the point in clinging
onto Socialist ideals when everybody is just lining their
own nest?' took over.

Let's party! And we did.

Struggling to find my feet once again in that crazy place
called London with no fixed abode and no fixed income,
I kind of skated, slipped and wobbled between Hackney
and Maida Vale where Jim lived. My drug sessions were
taken when and wherever they were offered, temporary
escapes from the stress of the reality I'd created for
myself. I think in the back of my mind I must have
known and accepted that I was in this situation because
I'd put myself there but I couldn't admit it then because
every minute of the day was permanent stress, a question

mark over my head as the only response to questions like: 'What happens next?' and 'What are you going to do now?'

Something inside me had been beaten irreparably out of shape – talent perhaps, belief in my talent – definitely. I couldn't find the inner strength to claw my way back to a stable place where I might take stock and find a way out of the downward spiral I was in. I couldn't see that at the time though and just kept on using drugs and drink to cushion the blows and it was through Jim's new social world in and around Maida Vale that I had my first experience of Ecstasy.

18 - Matches

Matches are not a new invention. There are records of 'the light-bringing slave' as it was known in 14th century China - small sticks of pinewood with their tips dipped in sulphur and taking combustion from other naked flames. Early matches did not initially self-combust and a self-combusting match really was the major scientific breakthrough of their age – the ability to make fire with one gesture, an action capable of being utilised by every single human being on the planet and putting to an end forever the tedious, unreliable methods that dogged only our ancestors' daily lives. Almost everybody had about their person or in their homes a dry bag or box where very dry dust or tinder, such as dried hair, wood-shavings, dried leaves or paper, was stored. Somewhere in amongst that would be a stone or mineral capable of making a spark. Other methods involved rapid and repetitive abrasion of two pieces of wood with a simple supply of fresh oxygen in exactly the same place where the abrasion is concentrated.

After the discovery of the ability to grind certain materials to make glass lens, the 'burning glass' could also be used to concentrate the sun's heat into a single beam but this was only possible in the daytime, at certain times and yet impossible at night or in cloudy or wet weather. The other option was to simply re-fuel an existing fire and to keep it burning for as long as possible, day and night, winter or summer but a more practical and cheaper alternative was the use of candles which were also kept constantly illuminated. Tallow candles were the cheapest and based on the composition of animal fats but the wealthier households used beeswax candles. Tallow candle flames burned erratically and rapidly whereas beeswax produced a slow and steady flame.

With the discovery of gunpowder, flints comprising pig iron and powder were used in flintlock pistols and rifles.

The burning power of phosphorus (from the stone phosphate) was first discovered in 1669 and further experiments developed using combinations of phosphate and sulphur but nothing of the simplicity of a match had yet been thought of.

Most tobacco was smoked in pipes and though the majority were made of wood, they were also available in kiln-fired clay, generally having long necks tapering down to a small bowl that could be comfortably held with the hand outstretched at a right angle to the body and not less comfortably with the hand up closer to the mouth. One way of lighting the tobacco was via a 'spill', a think wooden object that looked like a straw. They were usually kept near the fireplace in a home. There was also a 'striker'. To our modern eyes this resembled a pair of separated scissor blades but one of the blades was the flint stone and the other was the iron. Generally, the sparks' brief, glowing specks of iron would have to go directly into the dry kindling and then be blown on very gently to feed the existing heat. Other than that all fireplaces had iron tongs that were used to lift or turn coals in the fire and these two could lift out embers of wood or other burning material.

Various other inventors struggled and failed to produce something both practical and cheap until in 1827 a man called John Walker in Stockton-upon-Tees in north east England came closest. Walker was a chemist with a shop in the town which, only two years previously, had been the destination for the very first scheduled cargo and passenger service from the coalfields of the north western parts of the county via the wool-trading town of Darlington. Demands for rapid and practical time-saving devices sprang up. Diligent experimentation brought Walker to the conclusion that it wasn't so much the contents of the material that produced the flame but how to ignite? He hit upon the simple idea of supplying a small piece of folded card like sandpaper in each matchbox. It was later conceived around 1859 that fitting a sandpaper surface inside the matchbox risked igniting the matches at any time so the simple idea of putting the striking surface outside the matchbox caught on. Thus the user would be able to strike the dried sulphurous material against a frictional surface at any time, anywhere. Once the mixture ignited it then slowly burnt its way up the wooden matchstick a few inches long, extending the life of the flame by almost a minute. He concluded that a flame that burnt for that length of time could add fire to any combustible material, not just tobacco but fire kindling too. Not only did his 'fire stick' ignite things, it also bought Man sixty precious and valuable seconds of light and heat in what would otherwise be a black and cold world. A man could do a lot with sixty seconds of light and heat.

His early matches were composed of sulphur, sulphide of antimony, chlorate of potash and gum, all pummelled in a small bowl as druggists were wont to do when preparing their medicines and potions. The gum made the elements stick together when dried. The initial odour given off was noxious but he conquered this by adding a drop of camphor oil. Sadly though, due to the materials used and the time-consuming process involved, the production cost was high and so out of reach of most ordinary people though of great use to the steam engine operators and drivers on trains and in the collieries who were now able to save money not having to constantly feed fires with fresh coals or wood to keep them burning. Now they could extinguish fires when not being used and restart them again at any time they chose. Between

1827 and 1829 he sold these boxes to various parties both at home and abroad but they did have a nasty habit of sometimes sending off burning particles and starting fires. Walker did not patent his invention and returned to his initial trade. But the idea had already established itself and also in 1829 a Scotsman called Sir Isaac Holden slightly improved Walker's chemical composition and demonstrated it to his chemical engineering students at his college in Reading, Berkshire. One of his pupils showed the idea to his commercially-minded father Samuel Jones, another chemist based in London. Jones' development were called 'Lucifers' but these were shown to have similar problems to Walker's in that they produced dangerous red hot sparks

'Lucifers' were altered yet again by a Frenchman called Sauria who replaced the antimony sulphide with white phosphorus. In 1843 William Ashgard replaced the sulphur with beeswax, again reducing the pungency of the fumes and this was then replaced with paraffin in 1862 by Charles Smith. From 1870 matches (matches were made from small blocks of woods with saw cuts separating each splint but leaving the bases attached. Later versions were made in the form of thin combs with splints broken off when required) were fireproofed by impregnation with alum, sodium silicate and other salts.

The successful London match girls strike of 1888 at Bryant & May's match factory was a direct response to the increasing number of suicides, deaths and appalling disfigurements caused by 'phossy jaw' ('phosphorus necrosis') an illness that manifested itself in the mouths of the girls whose job it was to produce the matches and who came into regular breathing contact with the phosphate. Phosphate particles literally ate away human bone tissue, including the human jaws and flesh around the chins and cheeks. In a world with no medical insurance or employee protection, the female workers were cruelly disfigured and cast out of both the factories and society in general where they inevitably died of either cancer or starvation.

Phosphorus was still used by arms manufacturer though, specifically in grenades and bombs, but the safety match developed alongside the less safe phosphorus matches and the overall idea was to incorporate red phosphorus into the sandpaper which meant the combustible material on the tip of the match stick couldn't ignite without contact. It couldn't, for example, be struck on a piece of stone. The Swedish Lundstrom brothers developed this new invention and displayed it at the Paris Exhibition of 1855. By 1858 they had sold 12,000,000 boxes. Today, the striking surface on 'strike-anywhere' matches is composed of 25% powdered glass, 50% red phosphorus, 5% neutraliser, 4% carbon black and 16% is the binder. The match head is composed of 45-55% potassium chlorate and 20-30% siliceous (like silica, a heat-resistant compound used as an abrasive) filler called diatomite (a kind of connector inside the silica). Some also contain antimony sulphide. Safety matches ignite because of the extreme reaction of the phosphorus with the potassium chlorate in the head.

So, the next time you're out camping in the wood and need a fire to keep away the wolves and the bears, you have a simple way to keep them at bay and yourself warm without too much effort. Smokers too have an instant way to create the fire necessary to deliver the nicotine, just as the heroin junkie does when heating their heroin to liquefy it. The only downside of course is that the amount of matches that have to be struck to constantly feed pipes and cigarettes, the amount of exposure to dangerous chemicals by those who manufacture matches as well as the wasteful use of natural resources are all increased by smokers who in essence create this voracious demand. The need isn't forced on them. They do it willingly. So stick that in your pipe and smoke it.

19 - Rolling Papers

Cigarette rolling papers (or 'skins' as they are often referred to in English as they are as thin and transparent as human flesh) are made from 'rag fibres' such as flax, hemp, rice straw and esparto (Spanish/Algerian grass used to make rope, shoes and paper).

Early in my addiction and in a search for a cheaper form of nicotine delivery I switched from classic ready-made cigarettes in boxes to rolling tobacco and quickly learnt how to make good use of rolling papers to get my fix. The two methods both have the same end of course. Buying ready-made in a box uses more resources, such as cardboard and silver paper as well as cellophane wrapping. There is also the widespread incorporation of chemicals in the tobacco to make it burn hot and evenly as well as the plastics in the filter. Ready-made, box-bound cigarettes are packaged in handy, square shapes that are designed to fit comfortably in jacket and coat pockets as well as in bags and other right-angle shaped spaces in our daily lives to make transportation easier. The packaging too is often eye-catching and brand-association is a strong feature of marketing. Taxes on tobacco products are almost always high in most countries in the world but especially on cigarettes, less so for rolling tobacco. Smoking ready-made cigarettes is also a much 'cleaner' and more adaptable method of nicotine delivery than a self-rolled cigarette. Cigarettes can be lit virtually anywhere (except in water or in heavy rain) at any time due to the instant access to the mouth and thus the lungs and the combustible nature of the tobacco in the tip of the cigarette.

Rolling your own cigarettes is a messier affair but costs are lower than normal 'straights'. Cost is probably still the biggest advantage to an addict. Ready-made cigarettes are usually sold in boxes of ten or twenty though a few examples are known around the world of boxes of thirty. They are especially easy to smoke when driving, as many addicts who drive know, but opening a skin in the palm of one hand, adding just enough tobacco to enable the paper to be then rolled into a thin tube and for the gummed end to be licked and stuck down in 30 seconds is a tricky procedure for the uninitiated.

Prices between the two variants – ready-made or rolled – vary according to each country and the tax and import duties applied but it is certainly true that an average 50g pack of rolling tobacco can last longer than twenty cigarettes.

What do I know about the subject? Well, probably no more than you do but I found out that the world's most well-known rolling papers belongs to the 'Rizla' brand name which in turn derived from the French family of Lacroix. In 1736 they bought a paper mill and created the Lacroix Paper Company. Their first major contracts were through Bonaparte who gave them a licence at the end of the 18th century. Prior to that his solders had vandalised books and used their pages to roll their cigarettes. In 1865 the Lacroix Company changed the formula and used rice paper as the main material. The French name for rice is 'riz' and the first two letters of the Lacroix name were added to 'riz' and so the 'Riz-la' brand name was born. Rizla became the market leader after 1942 when it patented a successful experiment to add a gummed edge to one side of their papers which when licked with saliva sealed the tobacco into an airtight tube.

In 1883 the cigarette rolling machine was invented, another first from the Lacroix family. Their basic design is still in use in rolling machines today. The ZigZag brand of rolling papers introduced "interleaving" by which each rolling paper in a packet is folded so as to link it to the next paper and, in 1906, RizLa introduced the first flavoured papers (menthol and strawberry).

Nowadays rolling papers are available in a wide array of materials, colours, designs, flavours, scents, weights and sizes - some prefer the taste of rice papers, others prefer wood or flax, some prefer stiffer paper, others would rather have an ultra-thin, transparent burn, some like a thick gum strip and some papers with no adhesive strip at all - it all comes down to personal taste. But try as they might to take our minds off the bottom line reality, whether you smoke rolly or ready-made, you're still an addict.

20 – A bad groove - 1989-91

In 1990 I met some guys who lived in a squat on the Kensal Road and thought I might be able to get in there. It proved impossible but at one point, a guy from the squat and I broke into a council flat further down the road with a view to squatting it. It had a steel door but they'd left a tiny window open in the bathroom and we managed to squeeze through but we couldn't squat it in the end because getting the steel door off would have taken welding equipment and the risk of heavy or noisy work would bring suspicious ears and the cops. I'd noticed when we'd climbed in he had some ferocious burn scars on his arms and back and I asked where he'd got them. The Irishman, Liam, told me a story. A few years before, he'd been out in the Australian outback with his girlfriend, driving around in a mobile home, stopping whenever they felt like. They were both smokers so they smoked a lot of grass. One night they'd stopped in the middle of nowhere, off-road, and as usual got stoned, fucked and fell asleep. He woke in the middle of the night to discover the van in flames and just about managed to get them both out, but not before both had been badly burned. Without mobile phones or any way of contacting the outside world, he had to leave her in a bad state and despite also being injured, walk miles to the nearest main road, flag down a driver and eventually get an ambulance. By the time they got there, Liam's girlfriend was dead.

After he told me that story I stopped chasing the idea of getting a squat with him. I tried to understand how he coped and if it persuaded him to stop smoking afterwards, considering the price he'd had to pay, but he said it hadn't changed anything. He still smoked cigarettes and dope, more so now, as it was the only way he could get through the days or not have to deal with the memories.

Not long after, I ended up working five days a week during office hours for GG Management, a investment firm in the City, just opposite Liverpool Street Station in the same year. I was paid £200 cash weekly. In return I had to invariably wear a shirt and tie, mixed in with clean white t-shirts. I worked out of the Post Room up on the 12th floor of a glass block, twice a day steering a post trolley around the building, distributing parcels and letters or picking others up to post out and ten times a day I'd nip outside to smoke a fag and call it 'pleasure'.

The regular cash injection meant that I was able to get my life more stable in Clapham Common, but it also meant that from Friday to Sunday I forked out most of it on drugs and drink, either with Jim over at Maida Vale or Michael over at Hackney. Instead of being the sponger on the edge of the crowd waiting for the generosity of others, I was now able to buy my own place at the table and not only repay generosity but also meet other drug-takers. Drug-takers made contact with other drug-talkers so it was always wise to reinforce the network of dealers and contacts – you never knew when your regular dealer was going to disappear, get arrested or stop dealing.

Over the course of the months that followed I went to Amsterdam often, leaving Friday evening after work and returning either early Monday morning or late Sunday evening. The flight, hostel and coffee, food and drugs on top would generally swallow all I'd made in one mad binge, but that was okay because I could survive until the next wage came around but, having said that, it didn't always work out. At least working in a bar was slightly better because I could fiddle the tills to keep myself in pocket money and got fed with pub food. In the GG Clerical job I'd sometimes be so broke I used to raid the fridges in the works' kitchens for slices of bread and then a few days later be in Amsterdam living like a king and heading straight for the basement of the Bulldog Café in the Leidseplein. I held fond memories of the time I'd been there a couple of years before in 1989 hitching and busking, playing Glen Campbell and Little Richard songs on a guitar to survive.

Later that year of 1990 I'd then met an Australian lady called Angie in Clapham, who shared a flat with two gay guys in Battersea. Angie and I started an affair and so I moved into Angie's. All the time I'd lived with Angie I didn't pay any rent. My ego convinced myself that whether or not I was living with them, sharing their bed or fucking them, they were still going to be living there and paying their own rent. From this point on I started to turn into a serious twat, largely brought about by the lifestyle.

Angie found herself a job temping at the Main Reception at the BBC and instead of yours truly thinking sensibly like: 'Wow, this is a chance!' It didn't make the slightest difference. I still couldn't find the confidence in me to deal with the rejections that would surely come. I preferred the lifestyle of shit jobs, shit money, irregular living and quick drug fixes than dealing with the risk of being sober, sensible and, most importantly, strong enough to deal with rejection, as not all my dreams would find instant satisfaction. There would always be negative hits on that road. Having said that, a little voice in my head at some point in that period living in Battersea with Angie, said: 'You have do something useful with your life!!' So I quit the GG job as a way of kicking my own lazy ass. That was easy enough. But get back into serious acting? The problem with the office job at GG was that it was piss easy and well paid and would have been so simpler just to get on with it, but I hadn't come to London just to do that. But what?

21 - Lighters

With the increased focus on creating reliable, cheap, self-igniting friction matches during the 19th century, scientists, engineers and chemists also focused much of their attention to developing 'lighters' - portable devices that generate a stable and consistent flame by combining flammable liquids of pressurized gasses with a spark. Following the rapid development of the flintlock pistol and musket, many millions of ex-firearms that were irreparably broken down or worn out for their intended use were re-adapted by having stocks or barrels removed to become crude and ugly but efficient fire-starting devices. But the first real 'lighter' was probably invented in 1823 by German chemist Johann Wolfgang Dobereiner (1780 - 1849). His 'Döbereiner's lamp' marked the start of an era where fire could reliably be created in an instant. This device had a simple design – zinc metal reacted with sulphuric acid, creating flammable gas hydrogen that burst into flame when it met a sparks at the mouth of the container, but because the device was very large, hard to use and highly dangerous, it never managed to gain popularity.

However, the first significant innovation after 'Döbereiner's Lamp' came in 1880 with the 'ferrocerium' by Carl Auer von Welsbach in 1903. This creation enabled the birth of modern, small, portable lighters and its small flint could create a tremendous amount of sparks.

One of the first popular models of lighters came from Ronson in 1926 then, in 1932, 'Zippo' was founded and their legendary lighter immediately become an instant success. The first truly 'automatic' lighter came in 1926 from Ronson and by the late 1920's there were four main types of lighter in use.

Naptha (petroleum/solvent) lighters use a saturated cloth wick to absorb the fuel fluid and prevent leaks. An 'arc lighter' uses a spark to create a conduit between electrodes and ignition. A 'flameless lighter' uses an enclosed heating element which glows and is most used in prisons, oil and gas facilities.

What else? Oh yes, don't get them wet, they sometimes collect fluff in your pockets and block the flint spark and there's nothing worse for a smoker than having a cigarette between his lips and a cheap fucking Chinese lighter that won't light.

22 – The Gateway Hypothesis

I think a brief look at the 'Gateway Hypothesis' is probably overdue. The 'Gateway Hypothesis' is the theory that if a user freely takes one drug, either a stimulant or an opiate, they will be more tempted to experiment with others. Now, I know from my own experience that this isn't strictly true – I always tried drugs that seemed to offer me the chance to just about control them and not be controlled by them, but the line between these two theories – or the line between my theories – is fine and open to corruption.

'The Gateway Hypothesis' also states that 'cannabis use increases the probability of trying harder drugs and may exist due to social factors involved in using any illegal drug. Because of the illegal status of Cannabis, consumers are likely to find themselves acquainting with individuals using or selling illegal drugs. Utilizing this argument, some studies have shown that alcohol and tobacco may additionally be regarded as 'gateway' drugs; however, a more logical theory could be that Cannabis is simply more readily available than other harder drugs but in turn, alcohol and tobacco are easier to obtain than Cannabis, leading to the 'gateway' since consumers are most likely to experiment with any drug.

An alternative to the hypothesis is the 'Common Liability to Addiction' theory (CLA) which similarly states that some individuals are, for various reasons, willing to try multiple recreational substances. I can't speak for Jim and what his thinking was, if he had any, but I had a voice on my shoulder that often said: 'Whoa!' and sometimes I think he either had a voice on his shoulder that said: 'Give it a try and see!' or didn't say anything at all. I'll never know.

As for my experiences, consumption increased, despite the increase in poverty, in line with the sense of rejection, mistrust and hatred of anything that represented the Establishment, combined with the potent mix of being with other young people in the same circumstances, stirred in with milk and sugar.

By the time I leapt forward by five years to 1990 in London, I was lost, miles from the principled person I'd once been proud of being. It was a merry-go-round. I was on it and couldn't get off partly because I was still mixing with fatalistic people and friends with much the same mentality as the friends I'd had in Middlesbrough. I hadn't changed. Fear and lack of self-confidence got the better of me and I continued hiding in London's murky shadows.

So after I quit the GG office job in late 1990, I decided to start a new career selling advertising space into various half-legitimate publications, something that Jim had become remarkably good at. Now earlier, when I covered working in crappy jobs as a means to make money to fund a drug habit, you'd think anybody with half a brain would learn from experience and figure out a way to get wise, but I could see for myself how well Jim was doing so I figured if he could do it, so could I. I hadn't at that point quite realised that although washing dishes, working in bars and pushing trolleys in offices might have been boring and repetitive, it didn't mean I had to completely lose the moral compass, as I was about to do.

23 – Life on the run - 1990

I was still living in Kilburn but Michael was under pressure from his housemates to get rid of me. My continued presence put our friendship under stress.

I'd been at an Oxford Circus job selling advertising space and hooked up with a few other sales people: a Scottish guy, Sean, and a French girl and her boyfriend and all of us struggling with nowhere to live. The French girl knew of empty council flats out in Dalston that could be squatted so the four of us went up and found two flats vacant. The French couple secured one in one block and me and Sean took one in another block next door. I was to live like this throughout the summer of 1991.

We had no furniture. We had electricity, but no cooker, no kettle, nothing, and the balcony was a foot-deep in pigeon shit. At night the cockroaches came out to play and we had to grease the legs of the cheap beds we'd bought at a local junk shop to stop them crawling in with us. In the hot summer months, occasionally the water would get cut off serving all four tower blocks and outlying houses and then we'd queue up at stop-cocks in the street with hundreds of other residents, like in the Blitz. This was London in 1991!

Sean went off to Spain soon after to work in hotels but I wasn't going to stay all alone in that squat with no security. A few times I'd come home to find the door wide open as other squatters had been round looking for vacant flats. They just walked in and when they saw the bed and suitcase and toothbrush, walked out again knowing it was occupied so I moved in with the French couple for safety.

Life went on peacefully for a while but relations between us deteriorated and they asked me to leave so they could give my room to another French guy. I couldn't leave. I had nowhere to go and not enough money to get a place so we had to negotiate and learn to live together, but there was a lot of tension. The truce lasted until about October and then they both went back to France and left me alone in the squat, which was a relief but worrying as I felt even more vulnerable. Soon after, I cut my losses and moved in with a nice German girl called Suzy.

I was still seeing Jim and we continued to procure E's and cocaine, speed, dope and once or twice some acid. Of course we also both smoked like chimneys - that never changed. Suzy was accepting but she shouldn't have been. If she'd had any brains she would have told me to fuck off out of it, but she didn't. She wanted to experiment. A lot of people from all walks of life wanted to experiment in those heady days in London. Maybe they still do, I don't know anymore. If we had E's, she'd be included, if we had speed, she'd snort it with us, if we had dope she'd smoke the joints.

So in yet another blind and desperate stab at reclaiming my life and future, I flew out from Heathrow to Malaga on a one-way ticket. It looked like running away and it was. Despite my best efforts and despite living rent-free in Jerez, as my money ran out I gradually reduced my diet but instead of giving up wasteful things like cigarettes and drugs, I smoked more and ate less. My weight plummeted. By some miracle I managed to get a friend, a guy who worked for one of the big sherry producers in the region, to pay me for English classes with his daughter but I was hopeless as a teacher, unprepared. And still I smoked and drank and took drugs whenever they were offered and still my weight fell. I remember once counting out 100 cents in 1 cent copper coins, found down the back of a threadbare sofa to scrape together just enough to buy a packet of Fortuna cigarettes because at least in smoking I was able to keep hunger at bay. In the evenings I'd hang out in local bars, dependent on people buying me drinks (I always ordered strong ones so I could get drunk as fast as possible or drugs so I could sleep).

Christmas came and went, as did New Year. I rang Suzy and she offered to come out and join me and then get me safely back to London but I told her not to. Why did I do that? I still don't know. It would have been much easier. She would have saved me. She would have saved us. But I'd have certainly ended up back at being a lying salesman or working in a bar fiddling tills. By early January things were desperate. I had no way of getting back to the UK. I even studied a road map of Europe and toyed with the idea of hitch hiking back. At least if I could make it to Calais I'd have a chance of getting back across to London. London was still the best oasis for recuperation and getting my hands on funds.

In Jerez meanwhile I made a new friend, Xavier. We were the same age and had a mutual love of three things: drugs, women and dance music. He'd just lost his business, a partnership running a tapas bar in Jerez. Xavier had a modern flat near the train station and we started hanging out together, his curiosity about dance music, London and travelling grew. Like me, he had little cash but his widowed mother was generous. Xavier told me we'd go back to London, make some money, buy some new dance music then come back to Jerez and stay with him and the two of us would then spend a fortnight going round all the dance clubs in Seville and Cadiz selling the music. It sounded like a plan. I had no others.

24 – Trainspotting - 1992

In London I slipped back straight away into my old routine with Jim – we three went out to celebrate by dancing at Chaz's club getting wasted on a cocktail of acid, E and dope (consequent thirsts swamped by alcohol) and to fund it all I spent the best of three weeks working out of Victoria on the telephone, as-good-as robbing a couple of companies in Germany of hard-earned currency, enough to buy dance music with Xavier and the two of us flew back to Seville and spent a period of time known to Earthmen as a 'fortnight' but for us passed by in minutes in a blur of taxis, flashing strobes, techno trance music, hot chicks and endless lines of cocaine.

I think by this stage Suzy was getting fed up and who could blame her? Most women want stability. She wanted to settle down. The time was ripe, for both of us maybe to have kids. But there I was still running as fast as I could or as fast as the drugs or my illusions could carry me. I went straight to Kentish Town but Suzy wasn't there. She'd moved and left a forwarding address but the landlord refused to give it to me as Suzy had specifically asked him not to.

I also believe at that moment the bottom trapdoor of my life fell open and everything I knew or thought I knew about myself fell out, taking my guts and heart and soul with it. Everything I'd done, I'd done to myself. How could I possibly maintain any kind of order, honesty, tolerance or maturity in my life now that I'd lost this most precious of people?

So I decided to quit smoking cigarettes and taking drugs AGAIN. It was penance, redemption for wilfully destroying something beautiful through neglect. I had no way of backing up this bold claim with anything other than hot air but without the actions, it would remain that. I tried to smoke less but the cravings were too strong and to try to buy some time away from nicotine I even bought the tobacco substitutes 'Honeyrose' but smoking these blasts-from-the-past was like smoking autumn leaves through a toilet roll and smelled like it as well. I found myself stuffing one after the other into my mouth, craving the routine.

That was the first pointless part of the plan to try and convince Suzy I was capable of changing and winning her back. The second part was to get a job and make some money and the only way to do was to stop resisting being a lying salesman and BE a lying salesman, with both hands on the steering wheel. The final part of the plan was to find somewhere to live.

It didn't turn out as I planned (of course) and ended up spinning me off in all kinds of directions, but a man needs a plan or at least the basis of one so he can steer his life in some sort of mess. Trying to be the principled working class hero had caused me nothing but grief so I'd abandon it forever and be a businessman instead.

The Hawley Arms in Camden, built within the arches of the railway line and bridge that cuts across the High Street above the canal, was notorious. When Mobile Joe, our roving drug delivery dealer, wasn't available we'd have access to E's and cocaine at the weekend down at the clubs and if all else failed we had the Hawley for spliff. For the last six months of 1993 the pub's owner had access to the windowless warehouses under the railway viaduct arches at the back, accessed through one sole door. There were picnic benches and snooker tables lit by neon but the space itself was very dim. It was around these walls and under the arches the dealers lurked. The dealers in the Hawley would sell £10 bags of grass. The price was handy and easy to pay for – no fiddling about with change. The quality was reasonable but the weights were bad, but they were meant to be bad so that smokers constantly came back for more to spend more money. And we did, boy, how we did. Camden Town, they knew, was packed with young people with money to spend. Where Carnaby Street had once been the heart of swinging London, Camden Town had stolen the crown. Youth from all over the world came to Camden to taste swinging London 90's style.

It was from about this time that Jim and I began to lose track of each other as friends as he pounded that long hard road of harder drugs and harder drink and I pulled back, reining in the alcohol consumption and switching to dope.

I started seeing a French girl called Lulu. We both smoked of course! I'd been reading Irvin Welsh's 'Trainspotting' the previous year up in Middlesbrough when I'd gone for a break to get my head together. I loved the ending where Sickboy took all the money and fucked off to Amsterdam, totally burning his bridges so he'd NEVER be able to go back without his betrayed mates killing him, especially Begbie. Camden Town was a wasteland for drunks, pimps and druggies and thus a kind of heaven for me, crammed at weekends with tourists and dealers but I knew had to get away from that scene and get my life in some kind of order. The few months I'd spent in Teesside the previous autumn had given me just a glimpse of a creative life I'd almost forgotten, the one I'd had before I'd gone to London in 1985. Where was that guy? What had happened to him? Was he dead or was he just sleeping?

25 – Dignity by the bootstraps - 1996

Lulu and I made a plan. We knew that if we returned to London we'd fall back into the same routine and lifestyle we'd just managed to extricate ourselves from. Getting away from there and going down to Spain to clear our heads had been a really great idea and it had worked, we'd given ourselves a break and we could capitalise on that. We were both coming up to our mid-30's and figured we could just as easily go on pretending to be in our 20's, pretending tomorrow never comes. But of course it always does. We looked long and hard in the metaphorical mirror and then dared to suggest to ourselves we both had talents we were neglecting. It had been gnawing at me for ages by then anyway, the memory of how my star as an actor had been assured but I'd blown it through lack of life experience and confidence. Lulu'd studied Tourism in France but had ended up working in a pizza bar. We had to get back on the right road again. London would surely be the wrong road again.

In Teesside we found a damp terraced house to rent near Middlesbrough and we also found a dealer. Once or twice I might have even suggested to Lulu that we stopped smoking cigarettes and, if we stopped smoking, we'd also stop smoking drugs. That became the ultimate problem in the end – we were known as 'the smoking couple'. We could always be relied on to have something to smoke, so we attracted like-minded people. That wasn't to say they were all bad, weak addicts – there were a lot of non-smokers too, but smokers attract smokers, let's face it, it's a conspiracy. Drinkers like to drink with other drinkers. Heroin addicts like to shoot up with other heroin addicts. We all feel safer with our own kind.

Our next-door neighbour in the first house we lived in was known around town as a wild man among the town's toughs. As a neighbour he was decent and often invited us into his clean and well-decorated front room, one wall reserved for a huge tropical aquarium, but the fact that you might also see him in the middle of a scrum of fifty battling policemen on a Saturday night was another part of his character, a part of his past he couldn't escape as long as he lived in the town. He wasn't really a dealer but he knew the contacts and kept us regularly supplied for about a year. When we were short of cash, Lulu would usually knock on his door and get something on credit. He could never say no. He rarely said no to me either on account of her. Then one day I went round and he said he'd had to stop dealing for a while because the police had been round, so he gave us the contact he'd been buying off who lived up in another nearby town called Bishop Auckland. We phoned them and then went up there instead. Mick and Babs: he a local 'hard man' and she his 'moll' since they were both teenagers, and their two little kids. But that's another story.

26 – The Showdown – 2001

In late 2000, Lulu and I split up amicably for various personal reasons, none of them connected to our bad habits, and she returned to France where a short while after she was in the early days of a new relationship with somebody else that would go on to last about nine years. I stayed in the UK and started living with a new lady up in the City of Durham who didn't smoke and didn't take drugs and had an impressionable young son. I was keen at that stage in my life to live without drugs but to live without hash and grass also meant stopping tobacco. I couldn't be smoking around the house. As a prospective stepfather, I felt compelled to show responsibility and knew my actions had to be visibly seen to be done. But smoking dope and smoking tobacco went hand in hand.

So I started to read Allen Carr's book on how to quit and decided to give it a go. With the help of nicotine patches, after a few days I managed to wean myself off the physical addiction and soon stopped using them. It worked for a good while and by plunging into the responsibilities of family life I stayed off for a year and a half. But it was never to be permanent. I'd always known that.

I felt I had to personalize my addiction and turn 'It' into a separate entity. It helps to personalise this 'thing' to some degree so each of us can make little compromises to maintain an even keel. Sometimes It feels like it's in one or other of these places but sometimes it's in all three: brain, body, soul. 'It' is an unwanted visitor, a parasite kidding the host into creating dependency. It is the most lying, devious, sly, conniving, manipulative scumbag on the planet but having said that It was effectively telling me – no, *dictating* to me. In Its world the lungs, that did so much of the work of feeding the poison into my body, needed a break so they could recover enough to reclaim those poisons again a little way down the line. The point I'm trying to make is that I wasn't taking the decision to dominate It, chain It up, lock It in a box and throw away the key. I was simply ignoring It but It was still roaming free and taunting me. That's how determined you have to be if you're going to kill your addiction. If you're not as determined as that, as I wasn't, I was in fact stopping smoking for a while to fulfil what I presumed was the role of good father. The break would only be temporary and sure enough I'd drift back. All It had to do was snap two fingers and we'd be back to where we left off.

My new lady, Debby and her son Ludo and I, left England and moved to France where we lived for a few months shy of Christmas 2001 up until Autumn 2002. The first two months we shared the home of Lulu.

In France smoking is endemic. I could just as easily say smoking all over the world is endemic but it's only when you stop smoking that you realise just how much. Ironically, you can't see actually see it even when you're in the midst of it. My particular world back then in 2001, my French world, was dominated by about two-thirds of French friends who smoked, tobacco and/or drugs. But now, though I was trying to break away from that world, I was still maintaining social relationships with smokers who had no intention of stopping simply because I had. It wasn't as easy as I thought it would be, simply stopping and expecting the temptation to stop. Temptation was everywhere, not only people at parties puffing away at cigarettes. You think it's so easy. You just say: 'Stop!' to yourself and that's it, it's over. But it's not because you're still moving and operating in that world of smokers and an ex-smoker only has to breathe in the smoke of a smoker and the feeling of wanting it back in the blood is revived. Breaking a self-imposed discipline is a fast track to restoring an old habit so just rolling something into a cigarette paper, sticking it into my mouth and lighting it brought back a million familiar memories of smoking a million cigarettes and joints.

We returned to live in Gateshead about two months later for various other reasons and it wasn't long before I was buying ten of the cheapest cigarettes I could find at the local newsagent's and slipping out onto the back step of our flat for a smoke in an attempt to disguise the fact from my stepson that I wasn't foolish enough to return to my addiction - which of course I was. And then when I ran out of smokes, actually go through the rubbish bin to recover a few old stubs and roll them up into a small Rizla to squeeze one last desperate drag out of the remaining tobacco to fuel my ravenous addiction.

The Beast was back.

I'd stopped trying to hide it from my stepson. Dignity and pride is often the first thing you lose, having to admit you're not strong enough to stay away from a bad habit to a young kid who looks up to you and your strength as a man. Of course you feel stupid because you *are* stupid, but addiction doesn't give a fuck about such niceties.

Around 2005, my ex-wife and I split up due to my inability to provide a regular income. It wasn't connected to my bad habits but (she'd used some of them to get through some difficult times during our forced separation) but they hadn't really helped. Partly because of the drugs, partly because of the lack of work, partly because of the lack of income, partly for lots of other reasons my marriage failed and by September 2005 I was living in a council in a tower block alone. I was then in the direst circumstances I'd been in since living in London 20 years before and tobacco and dope were my only friends in those dark days.

27 – Emigration - 2006

In May 2006, I quit smoking again with the help of nicotine patches and lots of long, long walks. I stayed off for about eight weeks, cleaning out of my lungs. The most immediate effect is to taste food with taste buds that aren't laminated with tar. The gums emerge as pink and not grey. Your breath stops smelling – no more odours in your living space or on your clothes and you again start to feel the presence of money in your pocket. And tobacconists are that, effectively: dealers. There're more than quite a few non-smoking tobacconists prepared to sell you your nicotine injections and trade on your addiction, laughing all the way to the bank. But I had a smoke-free, two-month period, trying to get myself in better physical and psychological shape to not only orient my life but get the voyage underway. I did okay, lasting until about five days before leaving England and then I suddenly cracked, phoned a local dealer to line a stranger's pockets with my depleted funds in exchange for drugs.

I stayed in Middlesbrough for a week prior to going to France and that meant spending a few days with my old friend Pete. I couldn't imagine being in his presence, drinking tea and staring at the wall for long minutes searching for conversational points. I wanted the time spent with him to be full of ribaldry and laugh-filled madcap memories. I convinced myself that would be impossible without some dope. Mad really, looking back now. I had to be artificially stimulated.

In July 2006 I left England and moved to France with some compensation money from my divorce, determined to make a life. When I moved, smoking in cafes and restaurants was still permitted. For countless millions of French people and for me at that time, sitting in a café smoking and drinking coffee or beer was considered the highlight of daily life. Much rumination and contemplation could be passed staring into space, chatting, sipping small cups of strong espresso, drawing heavily on the tobacco and blowing the smoke out. Although this image is romantic and there's a strong temptation to feel nostalgic, the truth is it's still a myth. You can still sit in a café ruminating, contemplating, chatting to others and sipping from a small cup of strong coffee without pumping poisons and toxins into your precious lungs. The idea that doing so adds to the experience is part of the illusion propagated by 'It'.

I said before 'It' is a devious, cunning, fuck-face, right? 'It' will slip in by the back gate and ambush you and you won't even know you've been ambushed? 'It' never ceases to amaze, amuse and irritate me when I ask people why they smoke and they say: 'Because I enjoy it' but not comprehending that they're actually complimenting It. *They're* being smoked, *they're* being burned, *their* lives are melted down like candles.

A few months later I moved in with another lady - Lena - in a half-hearted attempt to find some stability, but coming so soon after my difficult divorce it was a mistake. She didn't smoke but I did. I stuck it out for about a year.

Those were hard days, those first months of being in France. The compensation money I'd taken with me didn't last long as I'd behaved like a tourist on holiday rather than a citizen eking out an existence and had spent too much, too quickly. On the other hand I was lucky and managed to get a teaching contract that paid well until the end of June in 2007, assisting a full-time French teacher of English in a school. Her name was Vero. Vero was a smoker too and yet I always felt stupid when she and I would stand outside the school gates at least three times a day, rain or shine, warm or cold, puffing away at our nicotine sticks and calling it 'fun'. If I wasn't doing that, I would be sitting in my girlfriend's car rolling one or two up and then going into work with professional people and trusting young kids looking up to me as being mature, sensible and wise yet reeking of smoke.

The new language challenges too were taking a toll and although a part of me wanted to go to dinner parties with French friends, another part didn't because inevitably I'd be linguistically lost, unable to follow conversations or offer opinions because they'd move too fast to translate. I'd flounder, grabbing whatever vocabulary I could to formulate an answer but by the time I'd translated it, the others at the table had lost interest. The worst was when somebody told a joke and everyone started laughing and

I'd be sitting there nonplussed. I had a hard apprenticeship picking up the subtleties and nuances so in fact it became actually easier, for that first year and a half, to drink too much and smoke too much and disappear into the silent world of my own head. Or at least that's what I told myself. The notion that I could actually take control of *my* life, *my* future, *my* health and *my* general spiritual wellbeing by NOT smoking seemed beyond me.

Other than that, I got through the summer by cadging off neighbours. Unable to find a regular dealer, I instead smoked far, far too many cigarettes.

28 – Big Effort - 2009

Cadgers and scroungers of dope are the lowest form of life and I was that. They hang around with those who have dope and pretend to be interested in their lives or make conversation where there are mere grunts, try to build links and bridges where none truly exist and feebly laugh at jokes in such a way that both parties know it's all a stupid game. If I was lucky I might get a couple of tokes on spliffs rolled or smoked in my presence but I was rarely able to get any of my own to take home and smoke. I had to have constant, vigilant patience, not my best virtue at that time. I don't know many smokers that do have patience, to be honest.

I struggled with cash through the summer of 2007 because the income had dried up and I'd no dole money nor regular work, so the only thing keeping me alive was the car boot sales over a dozen consecutive Sundays. It helped me improve my French and I made just enough cash to survive a little longer. I'd lost my marriage in England the year before partly due to the inability to provide any income and now, a year later, instead of being responsible and paying half of everything with Lena, I was being a selfish git and thinking only of my own comforts and bad habits. I'd come to France for a new start, to try to re-invent myself but the truth was I'd reinvented nothing. I was the same person living in a different place, back on hard times and desperate for anything to take my attention away from reality.

It was hard though to shake off the ghost of Jim and the ghosts of the people we'd been in those mental days in the early 90's in London. That was always what the point of drugs were for me – to get fucked up, to forget who I was if possible and to be so out of it that I could do anything I wanted and not give a damn. That's how it is in the world, in a way: we're programmed to behave and express through certain recognised social codes and patterns. But what happens when those patterns become routines? Drugs seemed to give me permission to do what I couldn't normally do. Despite not having lived in London for ten years and not having seen Jim for eight, there was still that residue of wanton wastefulness inside me trying to temporarily claw back that state of bliss I'd stumbled around with in London.

In a spur-of-the-moment decision I bought the nicotine patches and locked myself in my apartment for three days with DVD's and chocolates. Again, the physical dependence was quick to go and to get the toxins out I went out for three consecutive days and walked – no, marched – about 10 km. It was cold but I marched and marched, like a soldier on a long hike, maintaining a constant fast pace and not allowing anything to slow me down – not a zebra crossing, not a traffic light, not a busy road. I walked and walked and kept walking as my life depended on it, coming home knackered and sweating, giving my body a natural reason to sleep and not an artificial one. I was to maintain this state for over a year and a half, the longest period without smoking I'd yet been able to maintain. It was my second serious attempt to stop.

But there was still a Dark Angel I hadn't shaken off, sitting on my shoulder whispering temptation, risk, danger, and excitement in my ear.

There's not only a lot of talk but a lot of controversy these days over drug cocktails – addicts mixing different drugs at the same time in an effort to experience a new sensation or thrill and I have to admit that this was the case with me, not only as I'd done that night but as I'd done before in the past by mixing drugs. Anonymous people who merit only a few lines in a local newspaper's obituary column die regularly of these dangerous mixes just as much do the big name rock stars and film stars. There's a fatal flaw to all those humans who feel the need to take such risks, to push the envelope, search for short cuts to places where they feel they might chemically reproduce their Heaven on Earth, almost as if – despite all the wealth if they have any – they're still missing some element in their genetic makeup. But we weren't born with cigarettes in our mouths or drugs in our bloodstreams. We were born as nature intended us to be – clean and innocent and healthy, pretty much. All that we do, we do to ourselves.

29 – Relapse - 2010

For a whole year I was happy.

At work I no longer had to eat mints to disguise my foul-smelling breath. My smoking colleagues continued to take fag breaks out on the front steps of the school where I taught and I watched them in a strange way I'd never noticed before. I became a zealot once I reformed but I think that's quite normal and – for me anyway - goes hand-in-hand with passion. People would ask me why I stopped and rather than say obvious things like health and money, I'd say what pissed me off most was how utterly bloody pointless it was, how much I hated that there are no short cuts in life; we have to endure whether we like it or not because smoking or drug taking doesn't change one goddamn thing, not one iota.

In February 2010 another relationship ended and I stumbled and fell hard onto the rocks for a short while and reached for my crutch yet again. But if it's any consolation, anything I took was always after work. It was what I'd tried to impress on my teenage stepson:

first you have to do the work and make the money and then you can relax. But you can't smoke dope first and then do the work because you won't do any work nor look for any and you can't smoke dope and work at the same time. There's a simple order of things: work first and relax later. I doubt he listened, despite my efforts.

It was in part due to the failure of that relationship that from February 2010 I began looking for ways to move to Paris. Visiting the capital regularly and building a network, I was finally offered a room in a flat share in the 18th in Paris. A withdrawal plan was made to leave Angers and move to Paris in September 2010. The flat was offered on the basis that I wasn't a smoker.

On 19th September 2010 I was invited to a wedding of two friends in Maine-et-Lore, one village down from the village I'd first lived in back in 2006. Blow me down with a feather if I didn't start that day by going to the local tobacconists and buy a packet of tobacco, some papers and a lighter and start smoking again! Why? I think it was the first time in many months I'd felt tested in a social situation where standing around chatting to people was an important element. I also knew a lot of people I knew would be there and almost all of them were smokers. The little voice inside – 'It' – said: 'Fuck it. Go for it. You can stop again in the future when things get too bad.'

I began to wonder in fact if I had two little voices in my head – It tempting me to smoke and get fucked up, and the other – not yet christened - resisting and shouting at It and pushing him away. That evening I was there with all the other mugs puffing away on cigarettes offered to me and rolling my own like I'd never had an eighteen-month break. When people I knew who knew I'd quit and with whom I'd been zealous saw me smoking, I defended it by saying I'd always known I might slip back into it again and I'd a history of taking long breaks and letting my body recover. But it was a bit weak.

The ideal situation of course is not to smoke and get fucked up at all but we don't all live in an ideal world. My ex at that time was capable of smoking one cigarette and then not smoking another for a week. I'd been around her for almost two years so I knew that was true.

Why couldn't I exercise the same self-control? For me it was either do it full on or don't do it at all, no middle ground. Why?

30 – Stumbling in the city - 2011

I turned up in Paris the next day with a packet of rolling tobacco in my back pocket, every inch the image of what I presumed the cool average Parisian would be packing.

Temptation was everywhere. One Metro stop down from where I lived was flooded with dealers in anything illegal. The hash there was of variable quality and hardly any weight at all, yet always €20. The availability, relative cheapness and the fact that I was now smoking and back to my old habits meant that I was there regularly but it was high-visibility and high-risk and like most addicts I always felt a sense of 'It won't happen to me'.

At night I was living in a tiny room alone in a flat. I think prisoners had bigger cells. Going out for fun was tricky because life there was just so expensive. Of course it would have helped if I hadn't smoked and saved cash to allow me to go out more because it really came down to one or the other, not both, but once I'd fallen into the trap it meant getting out again was going to take a lot of inner strength I just didn't have. I was enmeshed in all the cloying elements that dependency produces: hard life, lack of friends, vulnerability, money to pay, easy availability, regular supply, bad quality and over-consumption. It was a classic.

In February 2011, me and the anonymous Arab-Tunisian dealer who sold me some 'shit' got arrested by plainclothes police near the Metro Gare du Nord in Paris and charged. I spent a few hours in a cell and was interviewed so told the police truth as I saw it and took the blame for creating the demand. Without my demand there would be no need for supply. They let me go home that night. Next day I returned and they told me I was being conditionally discharged. The Dealer was put on Remand because he contested every word the police put against him, whereas I held my hands up and said: 'It's a fair cop' and walked.

But "It" was still stalking me a good fifteen years after I'd recovered my lost road and destiny. Now that I'd progressed to being a teacher most of my students loved me for my conviviality, unconventionality and self-belief, but I was still reduced to sordid drug binges in my isolation, trying to rediscover sensations lost to me, or fill the vacuum caused by a lack of a constructive and creative life or lack of a family.

It was just after being arrested that I decided to quit Paris and return to the world I'd known in rural France. Paris was okay but I missed a less stressful and cheaper quality of life, the countryside and friends, so I saved some cash and secured myself some Parisian work contacts so I could still come back from time to time and do some well-paid jobs, stretching my skills and adding new feathers to my cap, or arrows to my bow, depending on whatever euphemism you fancy. I planned to leave for good at the end of July and return to Nantes to live, sharing a cheap room in a friend's apartment and looking for teaching work.

I passed a quiet summer with no drugs at all, only occasionally managing to cadge some grass off friends but mostly doing without and smoking far too many rollies.

31 – And still the battle goes on . . . 2011-12

I started bumping into Guy whom I'd met briefly on and off over the years but should have perhaps bothered to spend more time with as he was a perfect mix of half-English and half-French. Problem was Guy was also a heavy smoker of both dope and tobacco, so although on the one hand I thought it could be good to cultivate a new friendship, especially with someone with whom I could converse easily and in my own accent, there was also the added problem of spending time with another addict. Guy rarely had any cash and like most of the people I'd met over the years he became my middleman, taking a dope 'commission' as a tip for setting it up. As soon as that happened and I'd jotted down his mobile number and then programmed it into my own phone there was no stopping me (or It) and, sure enough, I started to accrue more cash from the well-paid Paris-based company where I was contracted so I was on the 'phone to Guy twice a week. The price varied between €20-30, though the dealer – a second generation Algerian born in France called Ali - never seemed to be able to make up his mind if he was going to treat me as a friend, a friend of a friend or as a complete stranger each time we talked or met. That decision would decide the price. Of course, profit made the decision and soon I was on a weekly €60 treadmill with a variable quality of dope that kept reality from the door for a while.

There was only a slight improvement with the relationship with Ali in that he finally allowed Guy to give me his direct number. There was this insane part of me that wanted to prove to everybody that because I had lived through all types of shit in my life I was the bad-est consumer on the planet. All Guy's friends were the same as me – single men with no work and no money, addicted to sitting around all day playing games and cards, pratting about on Facebook like it meant something and scoring dope when one of us could afford it or if we pooled money and shared it when it arrived.

I was coming up to 50 and what had I achieved? What had changed? 50 should be a magic number. It seemed like one, like a gateway or a milestone. My lungs had had enough but I still wasn't ready to abandon the wish to smoke dope and as long as I had that desire I knew any attempt to quit would be only temporary, especially with the number of a very regular and cost-effective supply of drugs-a-few-touches-of-the-screen-of-my-phone away.

32 – D Day - 2012

On 30th May 2012 I locked myself into my rural retreat with a box of 11mg anti-nicotine patches, some DVD's and far too many chocolate biscuits and worked the dependence out of my system in three days, not needing to finish the course of patches I'd bought from my local chemist. Before buying them, the Assistant Chemist insisted on my completing a document to record my 'consumption characteristics' so she could advise me on strength but I already knew what I wanted and told her so – I was a veteran at quitting by now.

For six weeks I cleared my lungs, coughing up the vilest oil slicks into the toilet or elsewhere, sometimes doubling over in a public street or on country paths, wracking my guts out, tears streaming down my face, tempting hernias, trying to get that shit out of me. Tobacco withdrawal is a sobering experience.

Over those weeks I continued to see smoker friends but had no difficulty resisting. 'It' was surprisingly silent for the first time in many years. I wondered why? Perhaps because I was having no expectations or perhaps because I was doing what ex-alcoholics do – patting myself on the back for every day I got through without temptation?

End of June I went to a big street party in the village on the other side of the Loire. The clearest memory I have of that night is of hundreds, maybe thousands, of people smoking and drinking and not dancing at all but almost all standing around like sheep. It reinforced my belief in having made the right decision to quit.

I bought a slim, stainless steel pipe. The pipe was to replace my rolled up cigarettes. I decided I was going to smoke dope neat and pure through a pipe, instead of smoking tobacco, that way, I deluded myself into thinking, I'd still get the benefits of a good dope hit without being addicted to tobacco. I bought it from a head shop in Nantes. It was short and made of soft wood and unscrewed into three parts for cleaning purposes. I also bought some tiny gauze squares that nestled in the bowl to ensure crumbs of hash or weed stayed on the upper side of the gauze and didn't get sucked into my mouth or lungs. I scored through my dealer Ali in

Angers and got started on the pipe. The hit is harsh because 100% of the toxins and THC goes straight into the lungs – no filtering or burning agent like tobacco. The immediate reaction of the lungs is to expel these intense fumes via a cough as the throat burns much hotter than with a normal hash/tobacco mix. However, being as pure as it is, the hit is powerful, whatever the quality of the hash.

This became my addiction delivery system for the next 18 months, give or take. I'd basically swapped one addiction for another, possibly worse, but didn't see that at the time. When I started the pipe my only concern was not smoking tobacco again. I held firm on that one. It meant that on a social level, with other smokers, I wasn't limiting my options and could still go out with smokers but not accept tobacco offered in cigarettes or spliffs. I was still 'part of the gang', part of the general ambience, without feeling totally out of the picture. There's that underlying fear of losing out on something, a feeling of not being part of the group and being pushed to the edge of the circle. It's a scary prospect when you've spent years in the gang. I think even at that point I'd begun to accept that for people like me there was no such thing as a halfway house and that if I ever reached a point in my life where I had to quit everything forever, I'd have to close down ALL contact with people from my past who continued to smoke, otherwise I'd fall again. A lot of people I know – smokers – can't do that, especially French ones where social etiquette and protocol sometimes overrides logic and common sense. They can't (or lack the courage to try) close down familiar friendships or contacts or simply move to a place where they'll no longer be tempted. I thought I'd paid a heavy price for doing that but as time passed I realised the price I'd paid was cheap, considering what I gained in exchange. But I seemed unable to go anywhere outside of my front door without being stoned or under the influence, driving as well as walking.

And all the great acting plans came to nothing as days become weeks become months become years. Maybe there is some stimulation and inspiration to be found in smoking dope and, for people with bad backs or crippling diseases, some temporary relief, but when you're an actor it doesn't help at all. Just as I drive badly when under the influence so do I act badly too. You need structure and self-discipline to audition and deal with the focus of the auditions and the rejections. I kept on wanting it to help, kept hoping it'd somehow take me into a deeper part of my imagination as yet undiscovered, but in truth I go into these places much better without drugs. I do a lot more writing too. Having dope handy meant I would sometimes sit down and write something, but my imagination would wander and I'd smoke and start telling myself I was a genius anyway, regardless of the fact I had nothing to show for my noble claims.

I think I'd probably even soberly told myself: 'This can't go on forever. You have to stop.' But what would the catalyst be to force my hand? Partly it was age but I think there was also some sense of being locked in mortal combat with It and there could be only outcome. It would force me to feed it until the host body was lifeless and only then would the addiction stop, when there was nothing else to feed It. You can't feed death. It had all the characteristics of a suicide bomber. I had to beat It. I had to kill It but I knew I could never remove It because it was inside me. It was inside everyone. But each person fights their own battles in their own way and I had to have the strength to fight mine, beat it, lock It up under lock and key and never let It out again.

Addiction is a decision in the mind to be dependent and that was my recurring problem. I had to take another decision that said point-blank: STOP - not because of health or money or pride, though obviously these could be factored into the equation. I couldn't use them as primary, secondary or tertiary excuses. I had to associate myself with all those other billions of ordinary people in the world who got through life without getting stoned or drunk. There are a lot of smokers, stoners and drinkers in the world, that's true. But there are also an awful lot who don't take short cuts in life or seek them and just 'get on with it'. I have to admit, spending a lifetime, day in day out, just 'getting on with it' scared the shit out of me because it just seemed so dull, predictable, normal and *ordinary* and I'd pretty much lived my life being stoned under the illusion (or creating the illusion) that I wasn't ordinary.

There had probably been yet another little voice in my head in those early days in the 1980's that said: 'One day you'll have to stop but you can have fun until that day comes' and now the voice was back with increasing frequency, asking: 'Has the day come?' I was either going to have to honour that deal I made with my inner demon or become a permanent slave. Or dead.

One thing about being busy teaching was that I didn't spend too much time at home getting bored and looking for ways to occupy that time with the illusion of being busy. People who occupy their time with the illusion of being busy are people who, for example, call being on Facebook 'busy'. When I compared myself to Guy, I saw what would be in store for me if I had no skills and thus no quality of work to offer the world. In turn, no money meant a gruelling reality and the world is full of ways in which to avoid that gruelling reality. This usually involves sitting around rolling cigarettes or joints, smoking them and staring into space as if that's being busy. I see people everyday hanging around on the pavements outside cafes puffing away as if that action in itself is 'doing something useful with one's time'. Okay, maybe they don't consider themselves to be losers because they work hard and feed their families and do jobs that save lives or help people, but their fatal flaw is they're slaves to legal addictions. So using this definition, I'd become a loser and had been hanging out with losers all my life, on and off. I didn't want to do it anymore. I wanted to be happy with my own company, happy to live alone and be at peace with myself, accept myself as I was and live with that person, not despise that person or consider him dull or boring and feel the need to invigorate him with stimulants, like some fucked up hippy vampire needing a fix to come to life again.

33 – At last - 2018

It was only through a loving relationship that I was going to really find fulfilment as a human being, not through the sordid excesses of drug abuse that offered a gradual demeaning of self-respect and a long, slow degradation of the Self. When things got difficult in a relationship in the past, as a druggy I'd just turn around and walk away, knowing I could get fucked up so I wouldn't have to think about it or deal with it. But you *have* to love and respect yourself or you might as well jump off a bridge or under a train. Love hurts is the title of many a song about broken hearts. When you have love anything seems possible but it's not a gift that falls into your lap: you have to look after it and in doing so you have to look after yourself because if you're in no fit shape, how are you ever going to make an effort to love somebody else? It was easier to hurt myself and seek temporary and illusory short-term satisfaction in abuse than deal with the hurt. It's happened to me about half a dozen times now over my life – loving someone, losing them and then having great difficulties coming to terms with the sudden absence of love, filling the vacuum with mistrust, self-hate and abuse.

I was starting to understand I lived life for me, not for other people's expectations. I had to do something with my time, so why not that? I seemed to have forgotten how once, many years ago in the early 1980s before I'd fallen into bad company and started getting fucked up, I'd spent hours reading Shakespeare aloud or for friends and strangers. It had been an immense source of satisfaction but now, entangled as I was with drug abuse, it had become a kind of irritating chore.

And when we ran out of dope? Same with smoking - you pass a point where you can count down how many more smokes you can get out of what remains and then a mild irritation, stress and depression follow. When you're seriously addicted it turns into a kind of abject terror, this idea that you might have to get through the next twenty-four hours without being fucked up. You don't want it to end. You want that state of artificial bliss to be permanent. That was the main problem – *is* the main problem - drugs provoke emotions artificially, displace natural feelings, jolt them forward unnaturally, leap-frogging natural connections, seeking short cuts to normal human processes, pushing aside virtues like patience and listening.

The catalyst for my Big Switch Off was two words: 'No compromise'. The question to my lover at that time was: 'Do you think we might see each other more often instead of your work and your friends?' and the answer was: 'No compromise.' That was the catalyst. Nothing more complicated or less sophisticated. All relationships need work, compromise, consideration or patience – choose your upbeat adjective. This one wasn't going to get any, which was a shame, but I knew what was in store: self-doubt followed by self-destruction. That was my pattern. It had always been my pattern. Unless ...

It started the last two days in November. No need for nicotine patches this time – I wasn't ridding myself of nicotine but of the THC in cannabis.

I woke every day an hour before dawn, wrapped up, put on my old boots and walked 4km ever day.

No more drugs. No more influences. No more bullshit. No more pretending. No more Mr Bad Guy.

I'd have a steep walk back up to the village, often arriving sweating, purging the toxins and panting for breath, coughing up filthy black globs of tar that had its tendrils wormed into every cranny of my body. I imagined tendrils like internal puppet strings riddling and burrowing into every part of me, starting in the lungs and working through inner organs, heart, intestines, kidney, liver, muscles, arms, legs, neck, hands, abdomen, stomach, guts, thighs, legs and feet – all infected by addiction, every nerve-ending repainted brown and black. Each morning I went walking without fail, sometimes twice, again in the afternoons, forcing my fucked body to sweat the filth out of my bloodstream and lungs through exercise. I worked out too, forcing 50 press-ups a day. My diet changed. I switched from chocolate and biscuits to fresh fruit and water. To fill my time, instead of getting stoned and playing computer games or dreaming I was a film star, I read.

And then I took another big step: I deleted Ali the Dealer's number from my own phone's memory. I now had no way of getting in touch with him directly without speaking to Guy. I was now an ex-smoker and could see zero reasons to continue our 'friendship' as he and his mates still continued to smoke and his apartment was always full of the smell and odour of it. To confound the situation, Guy suffered from bi-polar disease, a type of depression aggravated by excessive smoking. What kind of friend tolerated that? I'd been free for about a fortnight and went round there one day and walked into a room full of smoke and nearly choked to death, having to open a window and just thought: 'Fuck this for a game of soldiers' and so I left and never went back.

I realised at that point that was what I was going to have to do with all my friends who smoked: cut them out as harshly as if they were cancers. There was no halfway house, no compromise – not for me anyway. If I truly wanted to quit this thing and get on top of it I had to rewrite the rules to suit myself and if it hurt some people along the way (smokers of course) then that was the way it was. There was absolutely nothing I could say to condone their lifestyle choices as being sound. They were mugs. I was a mug. I stopped being a mug. They continued. I told them so in blunt words and they rounded on me and hated me for it, accusing me of being cruel but I wasn't being cruel to them, I was attacking their addictions. It was their addictions that responded to me with fire, not them, not their true selves. Guy threatened to bop me the last time I was round, thinking I was bad-mouthing his character but I wasn't. I was trying to help him and get him out of the fog he was in. I mean he suffered from depression for Christ's sake! You look in any medical book and it says the last thing you should be doing if you have depression is take drugs and drink and get fucked up, so what did that make me, what kind of 'friend' was I to go round to his space regularly and tempt him to smoke and take drugs with me?

Meanwhile, the dawn walks around the base of the village, along the river up to next hamlet and back continued, clocking up about 4 to 5 kilometres a day and maybe 100-150km over December. Some mornings there would be a hard frost on the ground and it was like stepping on sugared icing, hot breath billowing around me as I struggled up to the old chateau. Other mornings it would just be cold, consistent rain and I'd be up to my ankles in thick mud.

I stopped mixing with people I'd known before and going to the usual bars. If it was my intention to go through life in some isolation, and my already small French world would be shrinking even more, then so be it. I'd rather live day-to-day in a comfortable and sober place in my own head than in a room full of losers terrified to change the environment for fear of the reality they would find. I see excessive drinking and drunkenness now for what it is or at least for what I think it is.

I knew Christmas was coming. I wasn't going back to England. But where could I go that didn't have smokers? Nowhere was the answer. I had to stay in my flat on my own. I couldn't discuss these psychological withdrawal problems I was having with anybody. I couldn't talk about it in public on Facebook for example and I couldn't talk about it with my parents. And even if I could have shared it with a confidante, I'm not sure I would have because I'd have been afraid I was confiding not because I was serious about stopping but because I was seeking sympathy. That's not how it should be, cold turkey. To get the full cleansing sensation you really have to go through the grinder and accept that the reason you're on your tod at Christmas is that you've wasted too many years hanging around with drug-addicts and smokers and neglected the relationships that could have and should have mattered.

That's how I ended up alone in my flat on Christmas Eve - in 2013 - in France - on my own. I sat at my kitchen table and cried like a baby for about half an hour. Sobs came crashing like clichéd waves on a beach, ebbing and flowing, tears down my cheeks, the outpouring of over 30 years of pain. I wiped them away with the backs of my hands. I had done this to myself. I kept repeating over and over: 'I'm so sorry, I'm so sorry' like apologising to some part of my personality I'd betrayed but was still present in the room.

I went out for my walk at dawn on Christmas Day to 'purify' my soul and figured that although I'd spend the day alone, it couldn't get any worse. Every day from that day was a building block. There would surely be tests. I'd be confronted with day-to-day problems but they'd be the same problems everybody else in the world faced and if they could crack them without breaking too much sweat or having too much stress, so could I. I knew from that day on what I would go back to if I relapsed.

I possibly could have done better things with my life. I could have (and perhaps should have) utilised my talent as an actor in more constructive ways. But with little education, little etiquette, almost no self-discipline and insecurity and ignorance heaped on my shoulders, I was loaded with too much too soon. Instead of dealing with it I buckled and reached instead for the proverbial bottle (or joint) as my crutch and it stayed by my side, too close by my side, for the next 30 years of my life.

I kept up my daily early morning walks until mid-January when I rounded the corner one morning to find the Loire had risen and flooded the usual path, cutting access to the hamlet, so I took that as a sign that it was time to stop my walking therapy and I was over the worst of my withdrawal.

Alcohol *is* fucking potent. They never truly tell you that when you're growing up. It only takes a few sips of something alcoholic and your body changes in the space of seconds. Drinking more and smoking more doesn't make the body respond any better. Drink more and self-control becomes gradually more difficult, smoke more and nothing really changes because smoking doesn't change anything, not for the better anyway. We say to stressed people: 'Have a cigarette and calm your nerves' but that's the last thing tobacco is designed to do, calm you.

I remember the date - 16th June I got the text message: 'Jim passed away yesterday'. He was 52. I got off the merry-go-round twenty years ago but it took me another twenty years of relapses to rid myself of all the associated self-destruction, guilt and insecurities that had made me so susceptible and open to drug abuse in the first place. I'd been easily led and in an effort to fit in I'd thought ciggies and drugs would be the perfect short cut to this goal of what I wanted to be: the cool dude. Jim was the cool dude and he didn't need drugs to be that, only he couldn't see it. He went into that world and after a while could no longer remember the one he'd left. The world he'd walked into became the only world he knew. The world I'd left was the world that saved me, in fact it drew me back from the brink and instead of my life amounting to nothing at all, helped me claw back some sense, sanity and pride. His family had disowned him. His friends had disowned him but, unloved and unwanted emotionally, what had really killed him physically was lack of eating and over consumption of strong alcoholic spirits and eventually alcoholism and cocaine abuse.

In conclusion then, the title of this book is a bit of a misnomer in that there is no 'killing' involved and 'It' is such a vital part of who we are as humans anyway that though we tell ourselves we hate 'It', we need 'It' and the temptations 'It' offers in order to test ourselves. 'Taming' might be a better word to substitute for 'killing' but 'Taming It' has less effect as a title. I can't kill 'It' and couldn't no matter how hard I tried. I can only tame 'It' in the sense that I can keep 'It' under lock and key in a kind of mental cage. I perhaps employ the strongest verb possible in order to remind myself of the need for constant awareness against apathy or familiarity because as soon as the prisoner gets familiar with the Guard's routines, it starts to plan its escape, so I tell myself (in a loud voice in my head): enjoy the life you've won for yourself but be vigilant every waking moment!

It seems to be working, so far

34 – The End

This is the end, my only friend the end. The book is over. Remember the deal at the start, about not smoking as long as you're reading? Well, this is it, the end. So now what?